EDUCATION IN A COMPETITIVE AND GLOBALIZING WORLD

GRADUATE MEDICAL EDUCATION ISSUES

Education in a Competitive and Globalizing World

Additional books in this series can be found on Nova's website under the Series tab.

Additional E-books in this series can be found on Nova's website under the E-books tab.

Health care Issues, Costs and Access

Additional books in this series can be found on Nova's website under the Series tab.

Additional E-books in this series can be found on Nova's website under the E-books tab.

EDUCATION IN A COMPETITIVE AND GLOBALIZING WORLD

GRADUATE MEDICAL EDUCATION ISSUES

CAROLINE I. HANSEN
AND
JOSHUA A. WOOD
EDITORS

Nova Science Publishers, Inc.
New York

For permission to use material from this book please contact us:
Telephone 631-231-7269; Fax 631-231-8175
Web Site: http://www.novapublishers.com

NOTICE TO THE READER

Additional color graphics may be available in the e-book version of this book.

LIBRARY OF CONGRESS CATALOGING-IN-PUBLICATION DATA

Graduate medical education issues / editors, Caroline I. Hansen and Joshua A. Wood.
p. ; cm.
Includes bibliographical references and index.
ISBN 978-1-61122-902-8 (hardcover)
1. Medical education--United States. I. Hansen, Caroline I. II. Wood, Joshua A.
[DNLM: 1. Education, Medical, Graduate--United States. W 20]
R745.G87 2010
610.71--dc22
2010044728

Published by Nova Science Publishers, Inc. † New York

CONTENTS

PREFACE

Reforming medical education will be a key component in transforming the nation's health care delivery system from one that historically has focused on care for acute illness, at the expense of chronic condition management, coordination of care across settings and disease prevention, to one that values patient-centered care, quality improvement and resource conservation. This new and important book examines the challenging issues in today's graduate medical education.

Chapter 1- Over the past 50 years, the practice of medicine in the United States has changed dramatically. Successful medical innovations have increased the complexity of delivering care while, at the same time, the U.S. population is aging and becoming increasingly diverse and the prevalence of chronic diseases is on the rise. In 2003, an Institute of Medicine (IOM) report on these changes noted that "clinical education has not kept pace with, or been responsive enough to, shifting patient demographics and desires, changing health system expectations, evolving practice requirements and staffing arrangements, new information, a focus on improving quality, or new technologies." The Medicare Payment Advisory Commission (MedPAC), an independent Congressional agency that advises the U.S. Congress on issues affecting the Medicare program, asked the RAND Corporation to conduct an exploratory study of how residency programs are adapting their teaching to prepare physicians to practice within the current health care delivery system, based on interviews with Internal Medicine (IM) program directors.

Chapter 2- Spending an estimated \$9 billion in 2008, Medicare is the largest financial supporter of graduate medical education. Averaging almost \$100,000 per resident per year, Medicare subsidizes education and training for about 90,000 residents in more than 1,100 hospitals through direct and indirect payments for graduate medical education. To some extent, this federal support signals the societal value the Congress places on educating and training our physicians. Despite this spending, however, a number of reports and articles have expressed concern that our health professionals are not gaining certain skills they need to provide the kinds of care that will best serve the public's needs.

Reforming medical education will be a key component in transforming the nation's health care delivery system from one that historically has focused on care for acute illness—at the expense of chronic condition management, coordination of care across settings, and disease prevention—to one that values patient-centered care, quality improvement, and resource conservation. Our medical schools and residency programs need to emphasize a set of skills and knowledge that will equip students and residents to practice and lead in reformed delivery systems that work under restructured payment incentives.

Chapter 3- Our nation's system of medical education and graduate training produces superbly skilled clinicians while contributing to stunning advances in medical science. Yet, it is not aligned with the delivery system reforms essential for increasing the value of health care in the United States. Research discussed in our June 2009 report, for example, found that internal medicine residency programs had limited focus on skills such as quality measurement and improvement, evidence-based medicine, multidisciplinary teamwork, care coordination across settings, and health information technology. These skills are important for producing the health professionals we need for a high-performance delivery system—one that provides high quality, high value, and efficiently delivered services.

In: Graduate Medical Education Issues
Editor: Caroline I. Hansen et al.
ISBN: 978-1-61122-902-8

Chapter 1

HOW ARE RESIDENCY PROGRAMS PREPARING OUR 21ST CENTURY INTERNISTS?

Kristina M. Cordasco, Mariana Horta, Nicole Lurie, Chloe E. Bird and Barbara O. Wynn

SUMMARY

Over the past 50 years, the practice of medicine in the United States has changed dramatically. Successful medical innovations have increased the complexity of delivering care while, at the same time, the U.S. population is aging and becoming increasingly diverse and the prevalence of chronic diseases is on the rise. In 2003, an Institute of Medicine (IOM) report on these changes noted that "clinical education has not kept pace with, or been responsive enough to, shifting patient demographics and desires, changing health system expectations, evolving practice requirements and staffing arrangements, new information, a focus on improving quality, or new technologies." The Medicare Payment Advisory Commission (MedPAC), an independent Congressional agency that advises the U.S. Congress on issues affecting the Medicare program, asked the RAND Corporation to conduct an exploratory study of how residency programs are adapting their teaching to prepare physicians to practice within the current health care delivery system, based on interviews with Internal Medicine (IM) program directors.

We conducted semi-structured telephone interviews with a randomly-selected and representative sample of 26 allopathic and osteopathic IM residency program directors. RAND worked with MedPAC to identify priority topics to be included in the interviews. Topics fall into the domains of three of the American Council on Graduate Medical Education (ACGME) common program requirements: practice-based learning and improvement; systems-based care; and interpersonal and communication skills. See Table 1ES for definitions of these program requirements and a listing of included topics by requirement. In addition, we assessed two aspects of the infrastructure that supports teaching in these competencies: the care settings through which the residents rotate and the information technology (IT) being used in these settings.

For each topic, we asked directors if his or her program teaches its residents about this topic, through either formal or informal (experiential) curricula. If the program did teach its residents about that topic, we then asked the director to describe his/her program's training. Probes were used to elicit details. After asking about the topics in each of the three core competencies, the director was asked about facilitators and barriers to education in that competency. At the end of the interview, we asked if the director perceived of any additional facilitators or barriers to improving graduate medical education.

Key Findings

In the competency of practice-based learning and improvement, we asked about programs' curriculum in evidence-based medicine (EBM), using decision aids, and quality improvement methods. We found that all programs are teaching their residents to use EBM through conferences at which residents present articles from the literature; the majority of programs also have formal training in searching the medical literature. Most, but not all programs are teaching residents quality improvement methods, but the curriculum varies widely; specifically, some programs have residents collect, analyze, and act on their own data, while other programs present the data to the residents and have residents informally participate in system changes. As for the topic of clinical decision aids, although all but one program teaches residents about clinical prediction rules and most hospitals use clinical pathways or pre-printed orders prompting the physician in standard or guideline-specific care, this education is informal at most hospitals.

In the competency of **systems-based practice**, we asked about programs' education in patient care coordination, working in multidisciplinary teams, awareness of absolute and relative costs, and patient safety. We found that although residents in all programs gain ample experience coordinating patient care, the programs vary in the amount of, and approach to, any formalized training and IT support in this topic. Similarly, all the programs interviewed provide some experience working with multidisciplinary care providers, but while a few programs have formal multidisciplinary teams, more often the teams are semi-formal or informal. All but one director indicated residents are taught to be aware of the absolute and relative costs of diagnostic tests and therapeutic agents, but most commonly this teaching is informal. Two-thirds of directors indicated that their residents receive instruction, most commonly informal, in patients' share of medical charges. Finally, all programs educate their residents in patient safety issues.

In the competency of **interpersonal and communication skills**— defined as "the effective exchange of information and collaboration with patients" — we asked about programs' teaching in communicating with other healthcare providers, communicating with patients, communicating with special populations, and communicating about end-of-life issues and advanced directives. Several program directors emphasized that although they have formal sessions on interpersonal and communication skills, the main, and most effective, way that residents build these skills is through experiences and faculty modeling, mentoring, and informal feedback. Additionally, we found that two-thirds of the interviewed program directors have formal teaching in communicating with other healthcare providers and all the programs have formal teaching in communicating with patients. Most, but not all of the programs formally instruct their residents in cultural competency. Half of the programs give formal teaching in health literacy, but less than one-third provide formal teaching in using interpreters. Most of the programs provide formal teaching in communicating about end-of-life issues and advanced directives, and all directors indicated that their residents get ample experience in this topic.

We found significant variation among the programs in residents' experiences with **diverse care settings and models**. Of the seven university hospital-based programs, four have required rotations in community-based hospitals. Residents in six programs rotate through Veterans' Affairs (VA) hospitals. Eighteen of the programs have a required rotation with hospice or a palliative care service. Twenty-one of the programs have required ambulatory experiences in community settings; however, for most programs this experience is minimal in time and scope. Fourteen programs have residents perform home visits and 21 programs have a required rotation in which they experience or provide care in a nursing home or rehabilitation unit. Twenty directors reported that their residents have some experience with managed care settings and/or populations, but seven volunteered that it was a very small segment of their overall patient population. No directors reported that their residents have experience in designated medical homes.

We also found wide variation in the use of electronic medical records (EMR) and computer order entry (COE). Although all programs provide residents with some experience in using EMRs, only one program has a comprehensive EMR in both inpatient and outpatient settings and two programs have no electronic system in their primary outpatient settings.

Directors reported multiple factors acting as facilitators and barriers to improvement, including:

(1) **Information Technology:** Having a comprehensive, or nearly comprehensive, EMR system was cited as not only key in giving residents experience in using such systems, but was also referred to as sources of data for quality improvement projects, tools for reinforcing the use of decision-support and prediction tools, methods to coordinate patient care in both the hospital and outpatient settings, and sometimes links to patient education materials. This was the most commonly-cited facilitator and barrier.

(2) **Faculty Expertise and Time:** Almost uniformly, a "faculty champion" who spearheaded the development and implementation of a curricula was central in areas in which programs have well-developed formal curriculum. Additionally, general faculty competency, or lack thereof, was a common explanation for informal teaching being either strong or weak in various areas.

(3) **Characteristics and resources of the program's setting:** Directors described how the settings in which the programs are based can be both assets and limiting factors in their residents' education.

(4) **Institutional support:** Program directors varied widely in their perceptions of the support that hospital administration and other institutional leaders provide. Several directors described areas where hospital priorities aligned with educational needs but in areas where there was not this alignment, less support was evident. Overall directors viewed ACGME's leadership in, and regulation about, these competencies to be helpful in getting institutional support. Some

program directors spontaneously expressed concerns about GME funding, worrying that if funds for GME were decreased, their institution may be unwilling to continue its support of residency programs.

(5) **Competing priorities for resident time and residents' baseline knowledge and interest in these topics:** Time to teach these competencies competes with both education in other competencies and with the institution's clinical service needs, especially given increasing knowledge and skills an internal medicine resident needs to master. Further, work-hour restrictions have decreased the time by which residents have to gain these knowledge and skills. Several program directors expressed concern that if, as recent reports have recommended, work hours become even more restricted, the residency environment may become even less amenable to instruction in these competencies. Furthermore, resident baseline knowledge, skill, and interest in, these competencies facilitate or impede their educational program in these topics.

(6) **Scarcity of research in educational and evaluation strategies for these topics:** Several directors mentioned that there is a dearth of educational methods or tools that have been validated as effective for teaching residents these competencies. Furthermore, several directors explicitly cautioned against automatically valuing formally-delivered curriculum (lectures, projects, web-based modules) over informal curriculum, as much of these topics are best taught through the experience of patient care, with skilled faculty mentoring.

In summary, although IM residency programs are adapting their curricula to prepare physicians-in-training to practice in a demographically shifting patient population and evolving health care system, there is substantial variation in programs' approaches to, and implementation of, instruction in the topics of interest. For many topics, informal teaching through faculty role-modeling and patient- focused feedback and discussions is predominant.

In general, teaching in these topics remains inconsistent and far short from that needed compared to what is recommended by various expert reports.[4-9]Although directors varied in their enthusiasm for, and awareness of teaching methods in, these topics, they were, in general, supportive of improving curricula. However, as several program directors warned, these policy changes must be formulated so that teaching in other areas, particularly medical knowledge and patient care, are not negatively impacted. Also, heterogeneity in health care systems, settings, and residents also revealed the need for flexibility in graduate medical education policies.

In conclusion, these findings suggest that changes in graduate medical education funding policies, accreditation standards, certification exam topics, undergraduate medical education and investment in research of educational and evaluation strategies could have a significant positive impact on how well IM programs are preparing our nation's physicians to care for our 21st century population.

1. INTRODUCTION

Over the past 50 years, the practice of medicine in the United States has changed dramatically. Successful medical innovations have increased the complexity of delivering care, while at the same time, the U.S. population is aging and becoming increasingly diverse, and the prevalence of chronic diseases is on the rise.[1-3] In 2003, an Institute of Medicine (IOM) report on these changes noted that "clinical education has not kept pace with, or been responsive enough to, shifting patient demographics and desires, changing health system expectations, evolving practice requirements and staffing arrangements, new information, a focus on improving quality, or new technologies."[4] The Council on Graduate Medical Education (COGME), the American Association of Medical Colleges (AAMC), the Pew Commission, the Commonwealth Fund, and others have also highlighted significant gaps between the education that student and resident physicians currently receive and the skills they need to successfully deliver quality medical care to a diverse and older patient population with multiple complex chronic diseases.[5-9] In response to these calls for change, accrediting organizations of allopathic and osteopathic residency programs have begun incorporating new topics into curricula and accrediting standards.[10,11]

The Medicare Payment Advisory Commission (MedPAC), an independent Congressional agency that advises the U.S. Congress on issues affecting the Medicare program, asked the RAND Corporation to conduct an exploratory study of how residency programs are adapting to prepare physicians to practice by interviewing Internal Medicine (IM) program directors.[1] RAND worked with MedPAC to identify priority topics to be included in the interviews, which are detailed in Table 1. These topics fall into the domains of three of The American Council on Graduate Medical Education (ACGME) common program requirements: practice-based learning and improvement; systems-based care; and interpersonal and communication skills. In addition, we focused on two aspects of the infrastructure that supports teaching in these competencies: the care settings through which the residents rotate and the information technology being used in these settings.

Practice-based learning and improvement is defined as "the practice of investigating and evaluating the care of patients, appraising and assimilating scientific evidence, and continuously improving patient care based on constant self-evaluation and life-long learning."[11] Over the past several decades, successful medical innovations have increased the complexity of delivering care. This increasing complexity has made medical care vulnerable to problems in quality; studies suggest that Americans receive approximately half of recommended care.[12] Therefore physicians must be able to assess the quality of care they provide, and to implement system changes for practice improvement.[6] In addition, in order to achieve a high quality health system, physicians need the ability to synthesize, and apply to clinical decisions, the rapidly expanding and changing evidence base, using clinical practice guidelines and decision-aids.[13]

The second competency in which our topics were grouped is systems-based practice. Systems-based practice is defined as "an awareness of and responsiveness to the larger context and system of health care" and "the ability to call effectively on other resources in the system to provide optimal health care."[11] Not only has the complexity of medical care increased in the 21st century, but the complexity of the medical care system has also grown exponentially. Discontinuity in care has increased (within a hospitalization, at hospital discharge, and in outpatient care), while the proportion of hospitalizations related to exacerbations or complications of chronic conditions requiring longitudinal care has also increased. Therefore, physicians, whether they work in a hospital, a clinic, a long-term care facility, or other setting, must be able to coordinate plans of care, work with multidisciplinary support staff, and utilize systems ensuring patient safety in this complexity.[14,15] Finally, to counter rapidly rising health care costs and increasingly limited health care resources, medical educators should teach physicians to incorporate cost and cost- effectiveness information into treatment decisions.[16]

Table 1. ACGME Common Program Requirement Definitions and Topics Included in Interviews

ACGME Common Program Requirement	Definition	Topics included in interviews
Practice-Based Learning and Improvement	The practice of investigating and evaluating the care of patients, appraising and assimilating scientific evidence, and continuously improving patient care based on constant self-evaluation and life-long learning	• Using Evidence-based medicine • Using Quality Improvement Methods • Using Clinical decision aids
Systems-Based Practice	The practice of investigating and evaluating the care of patients, appraising and assimilating scientific evidence, and continuously improving patient care based on constant self-evaluation and life-long learning	• Coordinating patient care during hospitalization, across hospital discharge, and in outpatient care settings • Using methods for improving patient safety
Interpersonal and Communication Skills	The effective exchange of information and collaboration with patients, their families, and health professionals	• Communicating with other health care providers • Communicating with patients, including special populations and about end-of-life care

Competency in interpersonal and communication skills is "the effective exchange of information and collaboration with patients, their families, and health professionals."[11] Effective interpersonal and communication skills are important in 21st century medical practice given the changing demographics of the country—both in terms of aging and diversity—and the increased prevalence of chronic disease. Successful prevention and chronic disease care requires patient self-management as well as physician-guided care.[17] Yet, many patients have difficulty understanding how to manage their own care, especially those who have communication challenges due to poor health literacy or limited English proficiency.[18,19] Physician skills in cultural competency and cross- cultural communication are critical to the delivery of quality care to all patients, irrespective of their race, ethnicity, culture, or language proficiency.[4-6]

The settings in which residents gain experience, and the information technology (IT) being used in these settings, are critical components of the infrastructure necessary for achieving these three competencies. In order to be adequately prepared to practice in, and navigate patients between, various health care settings, residents need exposure and experience in diverse care settings.[5,6] To increase quality, safety and efficiency, physicians must become facile with the tools of informatics, such as electronic medical records, computer order entry, electronic sources of medical care information and guidelines, electronic and automated communications with patients, reminder systems, and IT-supported clinical decision-making aids.[4,6,23-25]

This report summarizes data collected via semi-structured interviews with 26 IM program directors. After detailing our methods, we report the findings of the topics organized into the three core competencies. Following the discussions of the core competency topics, we report on the programs' care settings and IT infrastructure. Lastly, we turn to reporting, from the perspective of the program directors, the facilitators and barriers to teaching these topics, before concluding with a discussion of policy implications. To give context for our findings, we also include, in the appendix, a review of a sample of medical school curricula, assessing the scope of teaching in the topics of interest and the settings for clinical rotations.

2. Methods

We conducted semi-structured interviews with a randomly selected, representative sample of 26 program directors. We first identified all allopathic and osteopathic IM programs using the publicly accessible residency program directory on the websites of The American College of Physicians (ACP) and the American College of Osteopathic Internists (ACOI), respectively.[26,27] We randomly selected 59 eligible programs,[2] stratified by those with allopathic and osteopathic accreditation. We additionally classified each program by region of the country, whether it is inside a Metropolitan Statistical Area (MSA) and by hospital type (Academic, non-Municipal Community-Based, or Municipal). We used the American Medical Association (AMA) Fellowship and Residency Electronic Interactive Database (FREIDA) to identify the number of residents in each program.[28] Programs were eligible for sampling if they had residents in the 2008/09 academic year and had graduated residents in June of 2008.

Table 2. Topics of Interviews

Practice-Based Learning and Improvement	• Evidence-based medicine searching the scientific literature to answer questions critiquing the medical literature and applying it to clinical decisions • Quality Improvement Methods systematically analyzing the quality of care being provided in one's own or a group's practice Implementing systems changes with the goal of practice improvement • Using Clinical decision aids
Systems-Based Practice	• Communicating and coordinating patient care: at hospital discharge among multiple providers in outpatient settings across provider hand-offs in the hospital • Using methods for improving patient safety
Interpersonal and Communication Skills	• Communicating with other health care providers • Communicating with patients communicating clearly about diagnosis and treatment plans engaging patients in shared decision-making - educating about self-care activities counseling to enhance adherence and/or behavior change • Communicating with special populations acquiring cultural competency communicating with patients with low health literacy working with interpreters • Communicating with patients and families about endof-life decisions and advanced directives
Care Settings and IT Infrastructure	• Caring for patients in: community-based hospitals Veterans' Affairs (VA) hospitals Hospice or palliative care services community clinics or private offices - home visits managed care medical homes • Information Technology using electronic medical records using computer-order entry

We sent three e-mails to the directors of sampled programs, inviting them to participate in an approximately 60-minute interview. Directors were asked to send a return e-mail or call to accept or decline the invitation. Additionally, directors of allopathic programs received an email from The Association of Program Directors in Internal Medicine (APDIM), and osteopathic programs from The American College of Osteopathic Internists (ACOI), encouraging their participation. For those who accepted, an interview time was scheduled and a second email sent containing detailed information about the interview and a list of the topics within the interview.[3]

Topics for the interviews are listed in Table 2 and the interview protocol is included in Appendix B. The protocol was developed in partnership with MedPAC, with probes for information that was of particular interest to MedPAC. In addition, we pre-tested the protocol with three current IM program directors and incorporated their feedback. For each topic, we asked directors if his or her program teaches this topic, through either formal activities or through experience. If the program director indicated that they do, we asked the director to describe the instruction in this area. Probes were used to elicit details.[4] After asking about the topics in each of three core competencies, the director was asked about enablers, facilitators, and barriers to their teaching in that competency. At the end of the interview, we asked if the director perceived of any additional facilitators or barriers to improving graduate medical education.

A board-certified IM physician familiar with residency education conducted all interviews. Each interview was audio-recorded. Based on detailed notes and after reviewing each audio-recording, using content analysis with techniques from grounded theory, we identified the range of methods and resources used for teaching residents in each topic area and the perceived facilitators and barriers.

3. Sample and Interview Characteristics

We identified 381 eligible IM residency programs: 320 (84 percent) allopathic; 45 (12 percent) osteopathic; and 16 (4 percent) with dual accreditation. As shown in Table 3, a greater proportion of IM programs are located in the northeastern states (36 percent) compared to southern (24 percent), midwestern (27 percent), and western (13 percent) states; nearly all

(97 percent) are located within an MSA. The majority of programs are located in community hospitals (61 percent), but approximately one-third are in university hospitals (37 percent), with the remaining 3 percent in municipal hospitals. Of the 290 IM programs for which FREIDA has data on program size, the number of residents per program ranges from 15 to 180, with a median of 51 residents.

Table 2 also describes the characteristics of the 59 eligible programs from which the director was invited to participate (50 allopathic and 9 osteopathic). Programs having both allopathic and osteopathic accreditation are on both lists, which resulted in over- sampling of these programs. Thus, of the 59 eligible programs that were invited to participate, 45 (76 percent) have allopathic accreditation only, 5 (8 percent) have osteopathic accreditation only, and 9 (15 percent) have both allopathic and osteopathic accreditation. Otherwise, as shown in Table 3, the programs randomly selected for invitations were approximately representative of the population of IM residency programs with respect to geography, being inside an MSA, hospital size, and hospital type.

Table 3. Characteristics of all Eligible IM Programs, Programs Invited, and Programs Interviewed

	All IM Programs (381)	Invited (59)	Interviewed (26)
Accreditation			
Allopathic	320 (84%)	45 (76%)	20 (77%)
Osteopathic	45 (12%)	5 (8%)	2 (8%)
Both	16 (4%)	9 (15%)	4 (15%)
Geographic Region			
Northeast	138 (36%)	21 (36%)	13 (50%)
South	91 (24%)	11 (19%)	4 (15%)
Midwest	105 (27%)	20 (34%)	7 (27%)
West	45 (13%)	7 (12%)	2 (8%)
Within an MSA	374 (98%)	57 (97%)	26 (100%)
Hospital Type			
University	139 (37%)	17 (29%)	7 (26%)
Community	232 (61%)	39 (66%)	17 (65%)
Municipal	10 (3%)	3 (5%)	2 (8%)
Number of Residents (median)	51	48	52

Twenty-six (44 percent) of the 59 program directors agreed to and completed an interview between November 25 and December 29, 2008. Three additional program directors agreed to be interviewed, but we were unable to schedule times to complete the interviews. As shown in Table 2, the programs of the directors interviewed resemble the characteristics of the 59 eligible programs invited, except that program directors from the northeastern states are over-represented and we did not have representation from programs located outside of an MSA. The programs interviewed ranged in size from 15 to 128, with a median of 52, residents. Interview lengths ranged from 44 to 89 minutes, with a mean and median length of 65 and 63 minutes, respectively.

4. Findings

Our results are presented graphically in each section (Figures 1- 4), with programs arranged randomly; however, each number represents the same program throughout the figures. When we arranged the data in order of program size, geographic region or hospital type, no patterns were observed (data not shown to protect program anonymity).

Practice-based Learning and Improvement

Within the competency of practice-based learning and improvement, "the practice of investigating and evaluating the care of patients, appraising and assimilating scientific evidence, and continuously improving patient care based on constant self-evaluation and life-long learning,"[11] we asked about programs' teaching in evidence-based medicine, using decision aids, and quality improvement methods. Figure 1 graphically presents the results. We found that all programs interviewed are teaching their residents to use evidence-based medicine (EBM) through conferences at which residents present articles from the literature; the majority of programs also have formal teaching in searching the medical literature. Most, but not all of the programs are instructing their residents in quality improvement methods, but this teaching varies widely with some programs having residents collect, analyze and act upon their own data, while in other programs the data is only presented to the residents and they informally participate in system changes. All except one program teaches residents about clinical prediction rules and clinical pathways or ordersets (pre-printed orders prompting the physician in standard or guideline-specific care) are utilized at most hospitals; however,teaching in these subject is commonly informal and IT support for these tools is not prevalent.

Evidence-based Medicine

All directors reported teaching their residents to use evidence-based medicine. Eighteen of the programs hold formal sessions on how to search the literature (e.g., orientation to common search engines, searching strategies). It is common for the institution's medical librarian to lead these sessions and then be available to the residents as needed for consultation. The directors in five of the eight programs not having formal sessions on search strategies have the perception that their residents are already very skilled in this upon entering residency.

All programs reported having regular "journal clubs" or "evidence- based medicine" conferences in which residents rotate in leading a discussion about one or more articles from the medical literature. Half of the programs (n=13) provide residents with faculty mentoring or assistance from an epidemiologist or statistician in preparing this presentation. At these sessions, after the resident presents the article, attendees, with faculty guidance, discuss the article, critiquing methods and judging its applicability to their practices. Half of the programs have additional lectures on critiquing the literature and/or the basics of medical statistics and eight give additional formal evidence-based medicine assignments, requiring residents to perform literature searches and critiques based on encountered clinical problems and to present the information back to faculty and/or co-residents. In one program, the residents have a special two-week rotation in which they are not involved directly in patient care but instead participate in daily rounds with a medical team, doing literature searches on relevant topics and presenting the information obtained back to the team.

Most program directors additionally felt that this topic is also extensively taught informally through daily interactions with faculty in the course of patient care. One director reported having done faculty development on this issue to enhance this informal teaching. One program annually sends its chief residents to evidence-based medicine seminars to improve teaching in this area.

Quality Improvement Methods

Quality Improvement (QI) can be broken down into two component parts: first, the systematic collection and analysis of quality data and then, based on that data, implementing system changes for the goal of practice improvement. We asked program directors about both aspects of QI.

All but one of the program directors described a mechanism through which all of their residents receive exposure to the systematic collection and analysis of data about quality of care. In 18 of the interviewed programs, every resident works individually or in small groups on a specific quality assessment or improvement project. In seven programs, the faculty or hospital administration collects and analyzes data on quality measures (such as Centers for Medicare and Medicaid (CMS) core performance measures) and then presents the data to the residents. In seven programs, residents collect or are provided with data specific to their own patients. In seven programs, the residents use or have exposure to chronic disease registries. Eleven programs have lectures specific to data collection and analysis and three use computer-based or internet instruction in place of, or as an adjunct to, in-person didactics.

Among the 18 programs requiring that every resident engage in an individual or small group project, approaches and resources vary. Four programs enhance resident engagement by having the residents choose their project areas, rather than having it assigned to them. Two programs have placed this project on a rotation (combined with systems- based practice teaching) during which residents are not responsible for direct patient care; one program has placed it within a specific ambulatory rotation that spans several months. Some programs have developed their own curricula in this area. Most often, these programs have a faculty member with a special interest in quality improvement, or the hospital's quality management department is co-leading this curricula. Four programs instead, or in addition, use the American Board of Internal Medicine's (ABIM) Performance Improvement Modules (PIMs).[29] These modules were developed primarily for use by post- residency physicians to fulfill recertification requirements in self-evaluation of practice performance; however, several of the modules have been made specifically available for use by residency programs. Another resource used by two of the programs is The American Osteopathic Association's (AOA) Clinical Assessment Program for Residencies; two community programs use web-based modules developed by university programs. An informal resource cited by one director is resident interaction with a large private group practice that focuses on quality assessment and improvement, so that residents have exposure to these methods being used outside the academic setting.

In the subject of implementing system changes, seven programs have lectures or computer-based instruction, and four have resident-led projects. Ten programs have a subset, but not all, of their residents involved in designated practice-improvement projects. More commonly, programs have informal teaching in this area by involving residents in hospital-wide performance improvement initiatives (e.g., soliciting suggestions or feedback and providing information on progress).

Using Decision Aids

All except one program reported teaching their residents to use clinical prediction rules (e.g., pneumonia severity index, pulmonary embolism prediction score, risk score for unstable angina, coronary vascular disease risk score). Six have specific lectures on these tools, but, more commonly, instruction on their use is contained within disease-specific lectures (e.g., the pneumonia severity index is presented within a general lecture on pneumonia). Seven programs electronically support these tools through direct links or calculators, either embedded in their EMR or through intranet links. Additionally, five directors indicated that although their institutions do not formally provide these resources, residents commonly have some of these tools on their personal hand-held computers or access them through use of the internet.

In twenty of the programs, residents use decision aids such as clinical pathways or order sets for common hospital conditions. In nine of these programs the hospital's information technology (IT) system supports these decisions aids; at one program, the IT system supports their use only when residents rotate through the associated VA hospital.

Program Number:	1	2	3	4	5	6	7	8	9	10	11	12	13	14	15	16	17	18	19	20	21	22	23	24	25	26	Total
Evidence Based Medicine (EBM)																											
Formal Session- Searching Literature	x	x		x	x	x	x	x	x	x	x	x		x	x	x	x				x	x	x				18
Journal Club/ EBM Conference	x	x	x	x	x	x	x	x	x	x	x	x	x	x	x	x	x	x	x	x	x	x	x	x	x	x	26
Lectures on Critiqueing Literature	x				x	x			x		x		x			x	x		x				x	x	x	x	13
EBM Assignments	x			x	x	x				x			x							x						x	8
Quality Assessment (QA) & Improvement																											
Have Lectures /Computer-Based Training in QA	x		x	x			x				x	x		x				x		x	x	x					11
Hospital administration collects, analyzes, and presents data on quality measures	x	x		x		x									x	x		x	x								8
Each resident works on quality assessment	x		x	x	x	x	x	x		x	x	x	x	x						x		x	x	x	x	x	18
Residents collect or are provided data on own patients				x		x	x			x			x					x				x					7
Use Chronic Disease Registries		x					x			x	x					x		x				x					7
Have Lectures / Computer-Based Training in Implementing System Changes	x						x			x			x						x					x	x		7
Each resident does project implementing system change	x						x					x						x									4
Clinical Decision Aids																											
Use Ordersets or Critical Pathways		x		x	x		x	x	x	x	x	x	x	x	x	x	x			x		x	x		x		18
Formal Lectures on Clinical Prediction Tools	x	x				x					x		x												x		6
IT Supports Clinical Prediction Tools		x				x		x		x	x		x	x						x		x					9

Figure 1. Findings on Formal Activities and Infrastructure For Practice-Based Learning and Improvement Topics

Program Number:	1	2	3	4	5	6	7	8	9	10	11	12	13	14	15	16	17	18	19	20	21	22	23	24	25	26	Total
Communication / Coordination of Care																											
Formal instruction in inpatient provider hand-offs		X	X		X	X	X				X	X			X			X	X	X	X	X		X			14
Faculty/chief resident supervise sign-outs									X		X		X	X						X	X						6
Inpatient Written Sign-Outs Critiqued	X			X		X	X			X								X									6
Computer-Based Tool For Sign-Outs		X				X	X	X		X	X		X		X			X		X							10
Formal Instruction in Discharge Coordination				X		X		X		X	X	X		X	X	X		X							X		11
IT supports Discharge Communication/Coordination	X	X				X	X			X		X		X		X	X			X		X	X	X	X		14
Formal Instruction in Outpatient Coordination	X							X		X		X			X	X				X		X					8
IT supports Outpatient Coordination	X	X					X			X		X	X	X			X	X		X				X			11
Outpatient IT enables sending of patient care tasks							X			X										X							3
Multidisciplinary Teams																											
Formal Inpatient Teams		X				X	X	X	X	X	X	X	X	X		X	X		X		X	X	X	X	X	X	19
Formal Teams on General Medical Service													X			X			X					X			4
Semi-Formal Inpatient Teams	X		X		X													X		X							5
Informal Inpatient Teams Only				X											X												2
Formal Outpatient Teams				X		X	X	X		X	X	X	X														8
Semi-Formal Outpatient Teams	X	X	X		X				X					X	X	X	X	X	X	X		X	X	X	X	X	17
Awareness of Absolute and Relative Costs	X	X	X	X	X	X	X	X	X	X	X	X		X	X	X	X	X	X	X	X	X	X	X	X	X	25
Lectures on Costs/Cost-effectiveness						X				X						X	X			X	X						6
Lectures on Patient Share of Costs				X		X											X			X	X			X			6
Patient Safety Issues & Methods																											
Lectures/Activity on Patient Safety Issues	X	X	X	X	X	X	X	X	X	X	X	X	X	X	X	X	X	X	X	X	X	X	X	X	X	X	26
Lectures/Activity on Theories/Methods of Patient Safety Assurance & Investigating Incidents						X						X	X					X		X						X	6
Patient Safety Project							X				X	X														X	4

Figure 2. Findings on Formal Activities and Infrastructure For

Systems-Based Practice

Within the competency of systems-based practice, "an awareness of and responsiveness to the larger context and system of health care" and "the ability to call effectively on other resources in the system to provide optimal health care,"[11] we asked about programs' teaching in patient care coordination, working in multidisciplinary teams, awareness of absolute and relative costs, and patient safety. Figure 2 graphically presents the results. Program directors in all programs felt that their residents get much experience coordinating patient care; however, the programs vary in their amount of, and approach to, any formalized teaching and IT support in this topic. Similarly, all the program directors interviewed told us that their programs provide some experience working with multidisciplinary care providers. While a few programs have formal multidisciplinary teams, more often the teams are semi-formal, or informal. All but one director indicated residents are taught to be aware of the absolute and relative costs of diagnostic tests and therapeutic agents, but most commonly this teaching is informal. Two-thirds of directors indicated that their residents are taught, most commonly through informal methods, what the patients' share of the charges will be. All programs instruct their residents in patient safety issues.

We additionally found that four of the programs have rotations specifically for teaching their residents in systems-based practice. On these rotations, in place of providing direct patient care, residents engage in health care system activities such as attending hospital committee meetings (e.g., patient safety, pharmacy and therapeutics), working with case managers to coordinate the flow of hospital patients, and working in the pharmacy or laboratory. Another program protects a half-day per week of resident time on ambulatory rotations for such systems-based practice experiences instead of teaching systems-based care on a specific rotation. Two programs, without such a rotation, require each of their residents to be active in at least one hospital committee, such as quality control, nursing liaison, or educational committees.

Patient Care Coordination

Although residents in all interviewed programs gain experience in coordinating patient care in the inpatient and outpatient environments, that experience is variable and the programs vary in their amount of, and approach to, any formalized instruction, as well as IT support in this area.

Almost all directors indicated that coordination of care involving provider handoffs within the hospital has become an area of increased attention recently. Eleven of the programs have specific lectures (commonly in orientation) on how to "sign-out" patients; one program uses a web-based module for this instruction, and two give their residents written materials to read. In six of the programs, a faculty physician or chief resident supervises sign-out sessions and provides feedback on the quality of the sign-out. In four programs, the written sign-out forms are intermittently reviewed and critiqued by the program director. Two programs have a formal system for peer-to-peer critique of sign-outs. In ten of the programs, the institution has provided a computer-based tool to specifically support the sign-out process. In two programs, on-call residents are provided with personal digital assistants (PDAs) or laptop computers with this software.

For coordinating care at hospital discharge, residents in all the programs work with case managers and/or social workers in communicating and coordinating hospital discharge. In one program, there is a specific nurse who assists the residents in this coordination. Eleven of the programs have formal instruction in this area, and many of these have case managers lead this instruction. One program administers a test to evaluate the knowledge its residents have obtained in this area. At three programs, charts are reviewed to assess the quality of the resident discharge summaries. To facilitate shared-accountability and enhance resident education in this area, one program uses a team-based approach to discharge communication and coordination in which each of the resident team members has a different role for discharge planning and coordination (e.g., communicating with social workers, communicating with primary care provider, etc) . At another program, residents rotate through a special "Discharge Team" that, separate from the primary team, takes the lead on care coordination and patient education on the day of discharge. While on this team, under the mentorship of the program director, residents learn about care coordination.

Although it was not asked about specifically, the main vehicle for inpatient provider communication with primary care doctors at most programs appeared to be the discharge summary and/or a shared computer system. We did not specifically ask about care coordination in transitions to long term care or rehabilitation services and this was not spontaneously mentioned by any of the directors.

The institution's IT system supports the communication and coordination of patient care at hospital discharge for 14 of the interviewed programs; however, the level and type of support varies. In some programs, this support is limited to dictated discharge summaries being made electronically available for providers in hospital-affiliated clinics. At two hospitals, notes are scanned into the computer system so that they are available at hospital-affiliated outpatient clinics. At five programs, the IT system assists in discharge medication reconciliation. Most comprehensively, in three programs, a summary document about the patient's hospital course is generated by the computer system and provided to the patient at discharge.

All residents have a "continuity clinic," in which they have a panel of patients for whom they are the primary care physician (PCP). One of the roles of a PCP is to coordinate the care of patients who have multiple providers (e.g., medical specialists, physical therapists, psychologists). Eight directors reported that their residents receive didactics or attend case conferences on care coordination in the outpatient setting. IT supports outpatient communication and coordination of care in eleven of the programs. This support is limited to electronic sharing of notes between providers in seven programs. In two programs with outpatient COE, the system prompts the resident to include appropriate information when referring a patient. In two programs, providers (both medical and ancillary) send patient-care related "tasks" to one another, specifically requesting that a note or lab result be reviewed or acted upon.

Working in Multidisciplinary Teams

All the programs interviewed provide some experience working in formal, semi-formal, or informal multidisciplinary teams.

In 16 of the programs, residents have exposure at least once to working in an inpatient formal multidisciplinary team, in which non- physician personnel, most commonly nursing, social work, or pharmacy, rarely a nurse practitioner, are assigned specifically to the team and participate in the team's daily rounds. Formal multidisciplinary teams are most commonly used only on subspecialty rotations, such as intensive care units, hematology/oncology services, and inpatient geriatrics units. In four programs, formal multidisciplinary teams are used on the general medical service. Five of the programs without exposure to formal inpatient teams do have experience working in semi-formal multidisciplinary teams; this means that although they do not do rounds together, there are regularly scheduled meetings between the residents and non-medical personnel outside of rounds. Two programs have informal teams only in which multidisciplinary personnel are available for consultation or are independently assessing the patient and discussing issues with the team as needed.

In ambulatory settings, eight of the programs give residents some, but often minimal, experience working in formal multidisciplinary teams, defined as having experiences in which the work of the resident and non- physician personnel (e.g., social work, nutritionists, pharmacists) is formally coordinated. Commonly, these experiences are on geriatrics rotations or if the resident co-leads disease-specific education classes or group visits. In programs in which there are no formal outpatient multidisciplinary teams, the directors (with the exception of one program) reported that the residents have multidisciplinary staff available for consultation—most commonly social workers and less commonly nutritionists, pharmacists, podiatrists, and psychologists—in their ambulatory continuity clinics.

Awareness of Absolute and Relative Costs

All but one director indicated that their residents are taught to be aware of the absolute and relative costs of diagnostic tests and therapeutic agents. The most common approach to this teaching is through experience during patient care and related discussion. Seven directors reported providing lectures specific to this topic. One director reported using the expertise of hospital utilization management personnel to deliver these lectures and another reported that the graduate medical education office had hired a person specifically for educating residents in this and related billing and coding knowledge.

Seventeen of the directors reported teaching their residents to know about patients' share of medical charges; seven programs have lectures or other exercises specific to this topic. The remaining programs indicated that their resident clinics are free or have a minimal "user's fee" and, thus, their residents do not gain experience in this area. For those getting this instruction, the emphasis and content is specific to the financial and insurance status of their specific patient population. For example, in one program, residents must know the basis for their clinic's sliding-scale clinic policy and in another, where most patients obtain low-cost generics at a local retail store, all residents know the costs of the different generics at that store. In programs with a larger proportion of insured patients, instruction is in insurance co-payment policies.

Patient Safety and Patient Safety Methods

All directors reported providing formal instruction in issues pertinent to patient safety (e.g., prevention of falls, proper patient identification). This instruction is done through lectures, monthly departmental morbidity and mortality conferences, program director meetings, or, in one program, through internet resources. Two programs supplement teaching with computer-based modules that residents are responsible for completing outside of duty hours. Only six programs, however, provide lectures on theories and methods of patient safety (e.g., standardization, root cause analysis). In one program, the residents spend time in the pharmacy to see how their computer orders are translated into the dispensing of medicine, how automated measures reduce medication errors, and how physician orders can assist or impede with these measures. Four programs have all residents engage in patient- safety mini-projects, investigating the incidence of adverse events (patient falls, hospital-acquired infections) or investigating root- causes of a particular "near-miss" or adverse event.

Directors reported that informal teaching in this area is also common. One director mentioned having done faculty development to encourage and improve the quality of the informal teaching. Six programs have at least some (but not all) of their residents participate in hospital-wide patient safety committees. Three directors mentioned that if an adverse or "near-miss" incident occurred on a resident's patient, or for those who have "administrative rotations," if there is an adverse event in the hospital while they are on that rotation, then that resident is directly involved in the investigation by participating in the root cause analysis or related activities.

Interpersonal and Communication Skills

Within the competency of interpersonal and communication skills, "the effective exchange of information and collaboration with patients, their families, and health professionals,"[11] we asked about programs' instruction in communicating with other healthcare providers, communicating with patients, communicating with special populations, and communicating about end-of-life issues and advanced directives. Figure 3 graphically presents the results. Several program directors emphasized that, although they have formal sessions on interpersonal and communication skills, the main, and most effective, way that residents build these skills is through experiences, with faculty modeling, mentoring, and informal feedback. Additionally, we found that two- thirds of the interviewed programs have formal instruction in communicating with other healthcare providers and all of the programs have formal instruction in communicating with patients. Most, but not all programs, formally teach their residents the skills of cultural competency. Half of the programs give formal instruction in health literacy but less than one-third provide formal instruction in using interpreters. Most programs provide formal teaching in communicating about end-of-life issues and advanced directives and all directors indicated that their residents get ample experience in this topic.

Communicating with other Health Care Providers

Although residents in all programs gain daily experience with communicating with other healthcare providers, 15 of the programs give formal instruction in skills for effectively communicating with other members of the health care team. Two programs do this primarily through a resident retreat on this topic, nine through lecture and/or role-playing exercises, three through interdepartmental panel discussions or meetings, three through web-based modules, and two through formal evaluation and feedback from nursing staff. One of the programs providing lectures includes content on conflict resolution. Four program directors mentioned having the nurses and other staff evaluate their residents on communication skills.

Communicating with Patients

All programs reported having formal sessions for observing residents as they are communicating with patients and then giving feedback on their communication skills. In addition, 22 of the programs have a formal curriculum on communicating with patients clearly about diagnosis and treatment plans. This is done through lectures and/or role-playing, standardized patients, web-based instruction, and/or videos. Delivering difficult news was an area commonly mentioned as being taught through lectures and/or role-playing. Two directors indicated formally soliciting feedback from patients about resident communication skills and providing that information, in summary form, to the resident. Five directors reported videotaping selected resident-patient interactions and then later, with faculty and/or peers, critiquing and discussing the video. Half of the programs have formal instruction in engaging patients in shared decisionmaking, through lectures, role-playing, standardized patients, or internet modules. In one program, the department has hired a clinical psychologist specifically for teaching residents communication and shared decisionmaking skills. In one program, communication skills, in conjunction with elements of systems-based practice and practice-based learning and improvement, are the focus of a special rotation, during which residents are not responsible for patient care activities. Seven directors of programs in which there are many international medical graduates (IMG) mentioned needing to occasionally devote additional time and resources to building the communication skills of IMG residents who have difficulty with their accents, language, or culturally-appropriate interactions.

All directors indicated that their residents gain experience in providing patient education. Seven directors additionally indicated formally teaching the techniques of patient education. A few program directors referenced instruction in the general subject of how to be a good teacher; although this instruction is more focused on how to teach medical students and junior residents, they indicated that it also contains principles applicable to patient education. In three programs, residents engage in a specific patient education project or activity, such as leading or co-leading a class to educate patients about medical conditions (e.g., diabetes education classes). In eight programs, the residents interact with and receive teaching from health or nurse educators. In fifteen programs, the residents use electronically available resources for patient education; in nine programs, the computer system provides direct links to these electronic resources. One program has a special "patient library" that the residents can refer the patients to through an "educational prescription."

Twenty of the directors endorsed teaching, formally or informally, methods to improve adherence to medications or lifestyle modifications. This is a topic of lectures in ten programs; one program uses standardized patients for this instruction. In one program, this topic is taught by a clinical psychologist.

Program Number:	1	2	3	4	5	6	7	8	9	10	11	12	13	14	15	16	17	18	19	20	21	22	23	24	25	26	Total
Communication Skills With Healthcare Providers	X		X		X			X		X	X	X	X		X				X	X	X	X		X	X		15
Communicating Clearly With Patients About Diagnosis and Treatment Plan	X	X	X	X	X		X	X	X	X	X	X	X	X	X	X	X	X	X	X			X		X	X	22
Engaging Patients in Shared Decisionmaking	X	X	X	X	X	X					X	X	X							X			X		X	X	13
Patient Education		X				X					X		X			X		X					X			X	8
Counseling in Adherence / Behavior Change		X				X	X		X			X	X						X	X					X	X	10
Cultural Competency	X	X	X	X	X	X	X	X		X	X	X	X	X	X	X	X	X	X	X	X	X	X		X	X	24
Using Interpreters							X			X			X		X					X	X				X		7
Health Literacy			X			X		X		X	X				X	X	X	X	X	X			X		X		13
End-of-life Communications	X	X		X	X	X	X	X	X			X	X	X	X	X	X	X	X	X	X	X	X	X	X		22
Holding Family Meetings						X					X				X		X	X					X	X			7

Figure 3. Findings on Formal Activities For Interpersonal and Communication Skills

Communicating with Special Populations

All except two directors indicated formally teaching their residents the knowledge and skills of acquiring cultural competency. A few directors mentioned that their instruction in acquiring cultural competency is specific to the cultures encountered in their patient population and not necessarily transferable into other settings. The most common method for delivering cultural competency instruction is through lectures; however, two programs use video presentations, one uses standardized patients, and one brings in community members to speak. Four programs with large proportions of IMGs also use the multiculturalism of their residents, asking them to take turns speaking about something from their own cultures.

All but three directors indicated that all their residents receive some experience using interpreters. In those three programs, their patient population is such that interpreters are rarely needed, although telephone interpreter services are available, and the residents are instructed in how to utilize them if needed. Among the other 23 programs, the extent of experience depends on the patient population. Eight directors indicated that their residents receive specific lectures in techniques on the effective use of interpreters. When provided, these lectures are often performed by the hospital's interpreter staff. In one program, the interpreters use a competency checklist evaluating residents' ability to use an interpreter effectively. One director noted that, although they had provided formal teaching in the effective use of interpreters when they used in-person interpretation, now that they have switched to an entirely phone-based system, he did not think these lectures are needed.

For communicating with patients with limited health literacy, all but three directors thought their residents get a great deal of experience in this area. Thirteen of the programs provide formal teaching in this topic: ten through specific lectures, one using a standardized patient, one using web-based resources, and one using formal mentoring when residents engage in a required activity developing patient education materials.

Communicating about end-of-Life Issues and Advanced Directives

In all programs, residents have multiple experiences communicating with patients and their families about end-of-life issues. Additionally 23 of the programs provide specific lectures, role-playing, standardized patients, or web-based instruction on this topic. Seven of the programs have lectures, standardized patients, or on-line modules on holding family meetings. Residents in all the programs receive instruction in talking with patients about advanced directives. The institutions of three of the programs hold multidisciplinary Schwartz Center Rounds,[30] during which health care providers convene to discuss emotional and social issues that arise in being caregivers in difficult end-of-life situations.

Care Settings and Information Technology Infrastructure

We found significant variation among the programs in residents' experiences with care settings and in use of electronic medical records (EMR) and computer order entry (COE). These results are displayed in Figure 4.

Care Settings

The care settings to which the programs expose their residents vary widely. Of the seven university hospital-based programs, four have required rotations in community-based hospitals. Residents in six programs rotate through Veterans' Affairs (VA) hospitals. Eighteen of the programs have a required rotation in hospice or palliative care. Twenty-one of the programs have required ambulatory experiences in community settings (private offices or community clinics); however, for most programs this experience is minimal in time and scope. Fourteen programs have the residents perform home visits and 21 programs have a required rotation in which they experience or provide care in a nursing home or rehabilitation unit. Twenty directors reported that their residents have some experience with managed care settings and/or populations, but seven volunteered that it was a very small segment of their overall patient population. In contrast, in one program all outpatients are managed care patients. No directors reported that their residents have experience in designated medical homes; however, five directors indicated that their clinics are working toward achieving this designation or that they believe their clinics have all, or almost all, the features of a medical home.

Electronic Medical Record (EMR) & Computer Order Entry (COE)

All programs provide residents with some experience in using electronic medical records (EMRs). However, residents in only four programs use comprehensive EMRs, including computer order entry (COE), for all or the majority of inpatient care. Residents in the remaining 22 programs use a partial EMR for the majority of their inpatient work. These partial systems range from those in which all aspects except progress notes are electronic to those in which the only electronic components are laboratory and study results. Seven programs with partial EMRs have COE. At two of these 22 programs, although the program's primary hospital has a partial EMR, the residents experience a comprehensive EMR with COE when rotating through an affiliated Veteran's Affairs (VA) hospital.

In residents' outpatient settings, seven programs use comprehensive EMRs with COE; in one program, the EMR is partial but has COE; ten programs have partial EMRs without COE; and in five programs, the main ambulatory care sites do not have any electronic records. Residents in two of the programs use electronic orders for prescriptions. In two additional programs, residents with continuity practice at the affiliated VA clinics use a comprehensive medical record system, with electronic prescriptions, but those residents at the non-VA clinic do not.

Only one of the programs interviewed has comprehensive EMRs in both inpatient and outpatient settings. Among the others, four directors indicated that their institution is phasing-in comprehensive EMRs, while the remaining reported that this process has been put "on- hold" or did not indicate that it is being pursued.

Reported Facilitators and Barriers

Six major themes emerged from program directors' reflections on facilitators and barriers to teaching in these topics and settings: (1) The presence or absence of IT; (2) the presence or absence of faculty expertise and time; (3) the characteristics and resources of the program's setting; (4) institutional support; (5) competing priorities for resident time and residents' baseline knowledge and interest in these topics; and (6) the scarcity of research in educational and evaluation strategies for these topics.

Program Number:	1	2	3	4	5	6	7	8	9	10	11	12	13	14	15	16	17	18	19	20	21	22	23	24	25	26	Total
Care Settings and Models:																											
Community Clinic or Private Practice	x		x	x	x	x	x	x		x	x	x	x	x	x		x	x		x		x	x	x	x	x	21
Home Visits		x			x		x	x		x	x	x	x		x		x			x		x	x		x		14
Nursing Homes or Rehabilitation Centers	x	x	x	x	x	x	x	x		x	x	x	x		x	x				x	x	x	x	x	x	x	21
Palliative Care/ Hospice		x		x	x	x	x		x	x	x	x	x	x	x	x					x	x	x	x	x		18
Managed Care		x	x	x	x		x	x	x	x	x	x	x		x	x		x		x	x	x	x	x	x		20
Information Technology Infrastructure:																											
Inpatient - Comprehensive	x	x							x				x														4
Inpatient - Partial			x	x	x	x	x	x		x	x	x		x	x	x	x	x	x	x	x	x	x	x	x	x	22
Inpatient - Computer Order Entry	x	x							x				x		x	x	x	x	x	x			x				11
Outpatient- Comprehensive		x					x		x	x				x						x		x					7
Outpatient - Partial	x		x	x	x							x	x		x	x	x	x	x		x		x	x			14
Outpatient - None						x		x			x														x	x	5
Outpatient - Computer Order Entry		x					x		x	x				x						x		x	x				8

Figure 4. Findings on Care Setting, Models and Information Technology Infrastructure

Information Technology

The presence or absence of IT was the most often-cited resource acting as a facilitator or barrier, respectively, for teaching in several topics. Having a comprehensive, or nearly comprehensive, EMR system was cited as not only key in giving residents experience in using such systems, but was also referred to as sources of data for quality improvement projects, tools for reinforcing the use of decision-support and prediction tools, methods to coordinate patient care in both the hospital and outpatient settings, and sometimes links to patient education materials. Furthermore, several directors commented that not having easily accessible information about cost was the major barrier to their instruction in this topic and a few suggested that a potential solution would be for their IT system to provide information and feedback on cost and cost-effectiveness.

Faculty Expertise and Time

Faculty expertise was also mentioned often as a key determinant of the quality and quantity of teaching in these topics. Almost uniformly, a "faculty champion" who spearheaded the development and implementation of a curricula was central in areas in which programs have well- developed formal curriculum. Additionally, general faculty competency, or lack thereof, was a common explanation for informal teaching being either strong or weak in various areas. Several directors mentioned that because some of these competency areas were not emphasized in the residency programs of many of their faculty members, the informal teaching currently being done is lacking, with some faculty potentially acting as "counterproductive role-models."

Programs vary in their ability to recruit, retain, and develop faculty with expertise in these competencies. For some programs, the institution and/or department have been deliberate about recruiting faculty with expertise in particular areas (e.g., palliative care, evidence-based medicine) and/or have had access to resources to invest in faculty development. Some institutions and departments require each of their faculty to develop an area of educational expertise, providing dedicated time, salary, and/or promotion incentives for teaching and other related activities. However, because smaller programs have a smaller faculty, it is more difficult for them to have faculty with expertise in all topics. Furthermore, program directors reported varying levels of influence over the hiring of faculty; one program director shared that at her institution, faculty hiring decisions are made entirely to fill clinical care needs, without considering specific graduate medical educational needs. Some directors expressed frustration that their faculty have insufficient time protected for teaching or to engage in faculty development in deficient areas.

Some programs have attempted to overcome their department's or institution's deficiencies through interdepartmental and/or interinstitutional collaborations. For example, two directors described partnering with other residency programs in their institutions to deliver formal instruction on communicating with other health care providers. Another program combines resources with other nearby programs and a local university to be able to provide videotaped standardized patient exercises in patient communication skills. One program funds its residents to attend lectures at a nearby university program. In developing curricula, one director in a community program described collaboration with the faculty of a medical school. Finally, some directors described informal collaborations, discussions at national meetings, ACGME's Educational Innovations Project (EIP), and email list-serves.

Faculty time was another commonly-listed key determinant for having formal curricula in this area. Several program directors described curricula that they would like to develop or enhance, but they or other faculty have not had the time protected to do so. (The programs do not have the funds to provide this time.) Many directors noted that because their faculty members already are implementing curricula in the continuously expanding medical knowledge curriculum, they do not have time to teach in these other areas.

Faculty time was also noted by some directors as a barrier to informal instruction in these competencies. Directors indicated that pressures to increase clinical productivity have resulted in faculty being less able to take the additional time to discuss issues with residents as they arise in clinical care Similarly, faculty now have less time to observe and provide feedback on residents' interpersonal and communication skills. Programs do not have funding to staff clinical sites with additional faculty who could focus on observing and providing this feedback

Setting

Directors described how the settings in which the programs are based can be both assets and limiting factors in their residents' education. For example, residents' experiences with diverse patient populations, and the nature of that diversity, are determined by the patient populations in their institutions.

Similarly, experience with different insurance and payment structures is determined by the institution and geographic area. Some directors reflected that their residents are practicing in settings that are "just not real world"; examples include having limited external pressures for productivity or cost-efficiency, working exclusively with uninsured or under-insured populations, having scarce infrastructure in ambulatory settings, and working with non-adherent patient populations. Thus, the residents are unprepared to work in other settings and/or have had such negative experiences with ambulatory care that they choose non-ambulatory specialties and practices.

Some programs attempt to overcome the limitations of their settings by giving residents exposure to community physicians. However, directors indicated that this has become increasingly difficult to implement in recent years as community physicians and organizations are less willing or able to absorb the cost of having residents in their practices. Two directors indicated that the program now provides small stipends to community physicians as incentives. Another program primarily uses its graduates for participation and thus depends on the personal relationships that the director has cultivated and maintained.

For some programs, models of care, resources, and patient populations are not available in their immediate community (e.g., managed care, patients who are culturally/linguistically diverse). Thus, to give exposure to these settings, program directors mentioned that a rotation away from the institution would be ideal. Furthermore, a few directors described how they thought away-rotations might be utilized for teaching quality-improvement methods or system-based care at institutions that have developed expertise in these areas. However, they reported that the current restrictions of Medicare graduate medical education funding are a barrier to setting up these rotations. If a resident rotates to another hospital, the home institution loses Medicare revenue for the time spent at the other hospital.

Institutional Support

Program directors varied widely in their perceptions of the support that hospital administration and other institutional leaders provide. Several directors described areas where hospital priorities aligned with educational needs, which meant that hospital development in this area was a key factor in the program's development in this area. The implementation of EMRs was the most common example of this alignment, but quality assurance and improvement, patient safety methods, patient care coordination, and multidisciplinary teamwork were also cited. Some directors reported that their institutions have been supportive of teaching interpersonal and communication skills by providing web-based learning and/or protecting resident time for building these skills, but more often the institution was less supportive of activities in this competency than in systems-based care or practice-based learning and improvement.

Although program directors sometimes disagreed with specific standards, they overall viewed ACGME's leadership in, and regulation about, these competencies to be helpful in getting institutional support. One program that is a member of ACGME's educational innovations project credited the requirements of that project as being key in getting increased institutional support. Another director, talking about the institutional support for teaching in systems-based practice, said "if there were a mandate, they would do it."

Some program directors spontaneously expressed concerns about GME funding. They worried that if funds for GME were decreased, their institution may be unwilling to continue its support of residency programs.

Resident Time, Baseline Knowledge, and Interest

Almost all program directors cited competing priorities for resident time as a barrier to effective teaching in these competencies. Time to teach these competencies competes with both education in other competencies and with the institution's clinical service needs. Several directors explained that in recent years the knowledge and skills an internal medicine resident needs to master, both in medical knowledge and these newly specified competencies, have grown exponentially. Yet with this increased volume of material, work-hour restrictions have decreased the time by which residents have to gain these knowledge and skills. Therefore, many directors noted that choices need to be made about the quality and the quantity of teaching in the different competencies and/or the structure or duration of internal medicine teaching. Several program directors expressed concern that if, as recent reports have recommended, work hours are restricted further,[31] the residency environment may become increasingly "fractured" and "chaotic" and, therefore, even less amenable to instruction in these competencies.

Several directors reported that resident baseline knowledge and skill in these competencies facilitates or impedes their educational program in these topics. In evidence-based medicine, several directors indicated that because residents enter with knowledge in this topic, all that is needed is a forum and structure for them to broaden their skills and experience. However, in topics such as quality improvement methods and systems-based practice, several program directors mentioned that their residents enter completely naïve to this area. In the words of one director, "it's a new language when they get to residency." (See Appendix for information on medical school teaching in these areas.)

Residents also vary in their baseline knowledge in interpersonal and communication skills. The need to do basic or remedial instruction in this area was cited often by directors of programs having a large proportion of IMGs. This remedial instruction sometimes absorbed a significant amount of program directors' time and resources.

Lack of inherent resident interest in these topics was also cited as a barrier. Some directors explained that their residents are more interested in the topics of the medical knowledge competency, because these are the topics that are tested in the American Board of Internal Medicine (ABIM) certification examination. Furthermore, the residents do not seem to appreciate how these topics will be relevant to their post-residency practices.

Research in Educational and Evaluation Strategies

Several directors mentioned that there is a dearth of educational methods or tools that have been validated as effective for teaching residents these competencies. Thus, directors called for increased research into curricular innovations with dissemination of results that would be easily accessible. Furthermore, several directors explicitly cautioned against automatically valuing formally-delivered curriculum (lectures, projects, web-based modules) over informal curriculum, because in their opinions, much of these topics are best taught through the experience of patient care, with skilled faculty mentoring. Finally, directors pointed out that it is difficult and time-consuming to evaluate their residents in these competencies, which hinders development and targeting of educational strategies.

5. SUMMARY AND DISCUSSION

In summary, interviews with the directors of 26 randomly-selected and representative internal medicine programs revealed that, although most programs have some teaching in the selected topics, there is large variation in the extent of and approach to this teaching and, in general, falls short from that needed, as recommended in several expert reports.[4-9]

Two areas of IM residency education stood out as relative strengths, in relation to the others: teaching in evidence-based medicine and communicating with patients about end-of-life care and decisions. Although IM programs vary in the formality of their teaching in communicating with patients about end-of-life decisions, directors generally felt that their residents gained ample experience in this topic. Secondly, evidence-based medicine is an area consistently taught through formal methods (with every program having a journal club). Program directors also have the perception that many residents enter with a good foundation of skill in this area; our review of U.S. medical school curricula (detailed in Appendix A) concurred with this observation as this topic is taught universally at all schools reviewed.

In both the IM programs interviews and the review of medical school curricula, teaching in evidence-based medicine and end-of-life communications emerged as relative curricular strengths. This may belie what one program director summed up as, "one does what one does well." Repeatedly, directors reported that teaching of evidence-based medicine and end-of-life communications is facilitated by having faculty members with expertise in these areas. This underscores the potential value of faculty development, or some other method of bringing to the program faculty expertise in the other topics, as an approach for improving teaching in these topics.

For many topics (both among IM programs and medical schools), informal teaching is predominant. The significant role of informal teaching, through faculty role-modeling and patient-focused feedback and discussions, further supports the importance of faculty development and ensuring that all faculty are competent in these areas. For example, even if residents are receiving didactic instruction in shared decision- making, but faculty role-modeling does not reinforce, or may even sometimes contradict, this teaching, then it will be ineffective. Therefore, it is not sufficient for programs to have a single faculty member with expertise in a topic, but also must ensure the basic competency of all their faculty members.

Although directors varied in their enthusiasm for different topics and awareness of teaching methods in these topics, they were, in general, supportive of improving curricula. However, as several program directors warned, any policy changes must be formulated so that teaching in other areas, particularly medical knowledge and patient care, are not negatively impacted. Also, heterogeneity in health care systems, settings, and residents also revealed the need for flexibility in graduate medical education policies.

In most topics, the teaching is inconsistent and, in general, remains far short from that needed, as outlined by various expert reports.[4-9] Most notably, the IOM's report on education of health professionals asserts that a core competency for health professionals is the ability to "communicate, manage knowledge, mitigate error, and support decision making using information technology."[4] Yet, only one of the interviewed programs uses a comprehensive EMR in both inpatient and outpatient settings and one-third have IT-supported decision- support. In the topic of quality improvement, few programs give residents experience with implementing system changes or teach basic safety design principles, as recommended by the IOM.[4] Few programs provide any formal teaching in using cost or cost-effectiveness in clinical decisions. The IOM additionally recommends that "most" patient care should be conducted in multidisciplinary teams;[4] however, only four programs have incorporated multidisciplinary teams into general medicine inpatient services. Experiences with multidisciplinary teams in outpatient settings are very limited or nonexistent. Less than one- third of the programs interviewed formally teach residents the techniques of patient education, a skill that is central to patient- centered care and essential for successful chronic disease management.[4,17] Furthermore, in contrast to COGME's recommendation that "clinical education should occur in settings that are representative of the environment in which graduates will eventually practice,"[5] residents in most programs have very limited experiences in community-based medicine or with working in managed care settings.

Given these marked deficiencies, we will now discuss our findings' potential implications for GME financing, accreditation bodies, the Internal Medicine certification exam, and medical school training.

Graduate Medical Education (GME) Financing

Medicare is the largest explicit funder of GME activities through payments it makes to teaching hospitals for the direct and indirect costs of teaching activities.[32] These interviews reveal several vehicles through which Medicare GME funding policies are affecting, or have the potential to affect, IM programs' teaching in these topics.

Graduate medical education financing is complicated because education and patient care services are jointly produced. Currently, GME support is provided through hospital revenues from patient care activities. In areas that experiential learning through patient care is the preferred method for instruction, this financing may be appropriate. However, program directors pointed out that, for curricular areas where didactic or learning outside of patient care activities is needed, this educational time competes with the institution's clinical service needs. The time spent by attending physicians and residents in educational activities reduces the time available for revenue-generating patient care activities and thereby impacts the institution's willingness to devote resources to educational activities. Furthermore, even in topics where instruction is patient-care based, faculty time to give, and resident time to receive, quality and comprehensive feedback, conflicts with the institution's service needs. As one program director explained, "Modeling is really important in medical education. And that just doesn't happen enough with people who are really good at this kind of thing because of time pressure on attendings and the residency programs . . . Imagine if you had the resources to have two residents per attending instead of four [in the clinics] and you had the funds for that? Then you would have time for modeling, feedback, etc. You would have a whole other level you could work on with the resident in these patient communication skills."

These interviews also revealed how GME funding formulas are affecting education in these topics. Formulas that determine GME funding rely primarily on the number of residents at a given institution and do not provide an incentive for institutions to invest in the quality of their teaching, faculty, or infrastructure, beyond that needed to attract sufficient residents to fill their approved number of positions. The interviews revealed how institutions respond to incentives in this area in that several directors conveyed how their institutions are more supportive of topics in practice-based learning and improvement and systems-based care, in which there may be gains in efficiency or quality indicators, compared to the topics of interpersonal and communication skills in which there are no such gains. Program directors expressed the desire for their institutions to have incentives to invest in their faculty's knowledge and skill in these topics through mechanisms such as: providing faculty development; prioritizing teaching skills in hiring, retention and promotion decisions; and finding alternatives to exposing their residents to faculty who might be "counterproductive role-models." Furthermore, payment mechanisms might be formulated to encourage informal teaching in topics for which this modality may be particularly effective (e.g., interpersonal and communications skills). Program directors also noted that their institutions do not have incentive to invest in outpatient settings; a prevalent theme was the relative paucity of infrastructure and formal curricula for outpatient, in comparison to inpatient, residency experiences.

Program directors pointed out that another way that GME funding policies are impacting teaching in these areas is by inhibiting rotations to other institutions. Some directors suggested that limitations in programs' settings, whether those limitations are in faculty expertise, community features or resources, or in the patient population, may be best addressed by utilizing rotations to other institutions. However, these directors also explained that Medicare generally only pays an institution only for time spent working in the hospital and hospital-associated clinics.[5] The hospital that is paying a resident's salary does not receive Medicare funding when a resident rotates to another hospital. While there is nothing to preclude the institutions from negotiating a mutually satisfactory financial arrangement, so that the home institution recoups the costs it incurs for the salaries of residents on away rotations, the negotiations are complicated by such issues as a limit on the number of funded resident positions at an institution and Medicare rules favoring resident time spent in patient care activities over time spent in didactic activities, particularly in nonhospital settings. These complications may prevent away-rotations that would enhance resident education. Addressing these barriers would be a potential target for enhancing resident exposure to diverse patient populations and settings and for encouraging institutions to collaborate and complement each other's strengths and weaknesses.

Accreditation Standards

These interviews also have implications for considering accreditation standards in these topics. Program directors reported that their institutions did direct resources to educational activities when changes in accreditation standards mandated or encouraged this investment. Therefore, standards that further encourage institutional investment could be synergistic with GME financing considerations. Furthermore, standards addressing the competency of the teaching faculty, and their participation in faculty development, could assist in addressing the major barrier, outlined by program directors, that much of their faculty do not have the skills to engage in effective informal teaching in these topics. Third, accreditation standards that further encourage experiences in diverse settings and outpatient skills may also enhance teaching in these topics.

The theme of competing priorities for resident time, and the ability to gather a sufficient mass of residents for didactic or other formal experiences, also interacts with accreditation standards through work-hour restrictions. Although patient safety concerns secondary to resident fatigue should obviously be paramount when considering work- hour restrictions, directors emphasized the potential negative impact further work-hour restrictions could have on formal and informal resident educational experiences on these and other topics.

Another implication of this study for accreditation bodies is the potential value of systematically collecting, in the course of accreditation renewal, data on the methods and success of programs' teaching in these topics. This data would give regular updates on the progress of graduate medical education, which could not only be valuable for policymakers, but also help with the program director's expressed need to have more research, data, and guidance for curricula development in these topics.

Specialty Certification Exam

Lack of resident interest in these topics may be a result of acculturation in the process of undergraduate medical education, or a reflection of the inherent interests of those who choose to go, and are accepted to, medical schools. However, at least some program directors felt that their residents were less interested in these topics because they are not present, or not emphasized, on the board certification exam. Although some of these topics may not be amenable to the standardized testing format of the certification exam, including them when possible may encourage resident interest.

Undergraduate Medical Education

Program directors' comments on competing priorities for resident time, as well as their observations that residents enter residency with differing or lack of baseline knowledge or skills in some topics, suggest the potential for improving instruction in these competencies in medical school. However, given that the current curricular strengths appear to be overlapping (e.g., evidence-based medicine, end-of-life communications), rather than complementary, much investment would be needed in further developing institutional capability and medical school curricula in these topics. Furthermore, although rotating medical students through settings outside of the institution does not have GME financing complications, and the institution is not dependent on students for clinical revenue, finding sites able to absorb the productivity loss associated with teaching students remains an issue. Furthermore, if this instruction were to be shifted from graduate to undergraduate education, a mechanism would be needed for ensuring these competencies in the 26% of residents that are graduates of non-US medical schools. Nonetheless, our review of medical school curricula does show that there are models for teaching medical students these topics that can be utilized as a baseline for developing medical school curricula in these topics.

Research

Program directors expressed a need for further research on the effectiveness of various methods and modalities for instruction in these topics, pointing to the importance of prioritizing funding for this research. Comparative effectiveness studies, evaluating the effectiveness of educational innovations, and developing methods for measuring resident knowledge and skills in these topics, would give the program directors the tools and data they need to improve curricula in these topics.

Limitations

This study was exploratory and its limitations should be considered when interpreting its findings. The findings should be interpreted only as a description of the range of current instruction in the various topics. Although we randomly selected programs, and the programs of the directors interviewed were approximately representative, on multiple domains, of the population of IM residency programs, given the small sample size and the semi-structured nature of the interviews, no inferences about generalizability or prevalence of curricula around a given topic can be made. A larger structured survey, informed by this study's results, would be needed to infer prevalences or differences by program characteristics (e.g., allopathic versus osteopathic, university versus community-based, etc.). Furthermore, this study aimed to gain a broad understanding of current Internal Medicine teaching in the selected compentencies. Each competency, and associated topic, could be the subject of its own study, gathering more detailed information on potential curricula elements and facilitators and barriers; if considering interventions targeting certain curricular components, in- depth studies should be done to inform that intervention. Similarly, case studies of programs and institutions that have been successful in implementing various innovative curricula would be informative.

Although, for clarity, this report assigns topics into discrete and non-overlapping categories, this portrayal may be both simplistic and somewhat artificial. For example, using clinical decision aids can be viewed as part of teaching evidence-based medicine, quality assessment and improvement methods are often taught in conjunction with system- based practice topics, and working within multidisciplinary teams is inherently linked with interpersonal and communication skills.

This study should not be interpreted as a study of the quality of the education being provided, but rather as a report on current methods being utilized. Programs with similar approaches and activities to teaching a topic may be delivering instruction at very different quality levels. For example, although all programs have journal club or evidence-based medicine conferences, the quality of those conferences may differ substantially between programs.

Similarly, as we do not know the effectiveness of various methods in achieving the various outcomes, we do not weight, or assign value to, the various methods or activities. Assessments of resident knowledge and skills, would be needed to measure effectiveness.

Conclusions

Exploratory interviews with 26 IM program directors reveal that substantial variation exists in programs' approach to and methods for implementing curricula in most of the topics of interest. In the topics of practice-based learning and improvement, although all interviewed programs are formally teaching their residents to use EBM, not all are teaching quality improvement methods, and among those that do, the curriculum varies widely. Instruction in clinical decision aids is informal at most programs. In the topics of systems-based practice, the programs varied in the amount of, and approach to, any formalized training and IT support in this topic. Few of the programs have formal multidisciplinary teams, teaching in absolute and relative costs is informal, and a minority have instruction on the theories and methods of systems to ensure patient safety. In the topics of interpersonal and communication skills, two-thirds of the interviewed program directors have formal teaching in communicating with other healthcare providers and all the programs have formal teaching in communicating with patients. Most, but not all of the programs formally instruct their residents in cultural competency but only half of the programs give formal teaching in health literacy and less than one-third provide formal teaching in using interpreters. Most of the programs provide formal teaching in communicating about end-of-life issues and advanced directives.

In general, teaching in these topics remains far short from that recommended by various expert reports. Directors report multiple factors acting as facilitators and barriers to improvement, including: available information technology infrastructure; faculty expertise and time; the program's setting; resident baseline knowledge, skills and interest; and, relative lack of evidence in educational methods and evaluation strategies for these topics.

Changes in GME funding policies, accreditation standards, certification exam topics, undergraduate medical education and investment in researching educational and evaluation strategies for these topics could have a significant and positive impact on how well IM programs are preparing our nation's physicians to care for our 21st century population.

Appendix A: Medical School Training in Selected Topics: A Review of Written Currricula

Introduction

Internal Medicine (IM) residency and all graduate medical education training builds on the skills and knowledge that physiciansin-training obtain in medical school. The degree of emphasis in IM residency programs on our study topics (namely, practice-based learning and improvement; systems-based care; interpersonal and communication skills) is influenced by the program directors' perceptions of the competencies that residents developed in these topical areas during medical school. To give context for our IM residency program findings, the Medicare Payment Advisory Commission (MedPAC) asked RAND to review a sample of medical school curricula to assess the scope of training in the topics of interest and the settings for clinical rotations. The structure of this appendix mirrors that of the main report.

Methods

We used lists published on the websites of the Association of American Medical Colleges (AAMC) and the American Osteopathic Association (AOA) to identify all U.S. accredited medical schools that have been enrolling students for at least four years.[33] We classified each medical school by whether it has allopathic or osteopathic accreditation, by region of the county by Census 2000 designations,[34] by being within or outside of a metropolitan statistical area (MSA), by being a public or private institution, and, for allopathic schools, by the tercile of grant funding from the National Institutes of Health (NIH) as reported on the NIH website.[35] Out of a total of 151 medical schools, we selected a random sample of 70 schools, stratified by allopathic and osteopathic schools and programs. Descriptive statistics of the above categorizations were used to verify that the random sample was representative along these dimensions.

For each selected allopathic medical school, we obtained the curriculum as detailed in the directory on the AAMC website.[36] For each selected osteopathic medical school, we obtained the curriculum from each school's website. We then reviewed the curricula of each school, identifying required courses and rotations that potentially included the topics of interest. We used the same topics of interest identified for the IM residency program interviews. We reviewed required courses only as we were interested in instruction that all the students receive, recognizing that students with special interest in some areas may pursue elective coursework. Courses were identified as being potentially applicable if they were not clearly focused on basic science or physical diagnosis skills. All "Internal Medicine," "Family Medicine," "Ambulatory Care," "Primary Care," and "Geriatrics" clinical rotations were selected when they were required.

We obtained email addresses for the person in charge of curriculum at each school through the AAMC directory and schools' websites. We emailed the contact person each school and requested syllabi and/or lecture topics for the selected courses and rotations at each school. We sent two follow-up emails if there was no response. We sent up to three reminder emails to those programs that responded that they would send materials. We assessed the curricula from all schools that provided syllabi or lecture topics for all of the requested courses. When needed for assessment of clinical settings, we augmented our data by searching school websites.

Sample

We identified 151 medical schools, 124 (81 percent) allopathic and 27 (19 percent) osteopathic. Table A2 describes these schools by geography, by public versus private, by NIH funding, and by being historically African-American. As also shown in Table A2, our stratified random sample of 70 schools was representative of the 153 schools on all these dimensions. We received syllabi and/or lecture topics for all selected courses and rotations from 26 (37 percent) of the schools. In comparison to the population of all medical schools, the schools from which we received curricula were more likely to have allopathic accreditation, be a public institution, and be in the middle tercile of NIH funding.

Findings

Overall Structure of Curricula

Traditionally, medical school curricula is divided into "pre- clinical" and "clinical" years. Pre-clinical years are typically the first two years, during which students learn the knowledge and skills that are the foundations of medical care through lectures, laboratory activities, and small group exercises. Then, in the third and fourth years, the "clinical years," students are placed in clinical care environments (known as "rotations" or "clerkships") and, with close supervision, learn to apply and build on this knowledge and skill set. However, medical schools are increasingly placing introductory patient care experiences into the pre-clinical years and some classroom-based courses in the clinical years. Accordingly, 17 of the 26 schools require a clinical "preceptorship" experience in the pre-clinical years, in which students shadow practicing physicians. Similarly, in 15 of the schools, classroom-based courses with variable topics are integrated into the "clinical" years. In some schools, these courses span an entire year, meeting one to two times per month, with students excused from clerkship activities for these classroom sessions. In others, these courses are concentrated into one or two weeks between clerkships.

The organization, detail, and extent of the written curricula received from the schools was highly inconsistent. At some schools, the skills and competencies that each student should obtain by graduation (sometimes mirroring the residency core competencies) are laid out and for each course, and there is a detailed description of how the course addresses these skills and competencies. For other schools, the objectives for each course were broadly described, without details provided.

Practice Based Learning and Improvement

Evidence-Based Medicine. The curricula of all schools reviewed have instruction in evidence-based medicine (EBM). Often, this instruction is in multiple courses spanning the preclinical and clinical curriculum.

Table A1. Characteristics of all Medical Schools, Schools from which Curricula Were Requested, And Schools from which Curricula Were Received

	All Medical Schools (151)		Requested (70)		Received (26)	
Accreditation						
Allopathic	124	(81%)	57	(81%)	23	(88%)
Osteopathic	27	(19%)	13	(19%)	3	(12%)
Public Institutions	70	(46%)	33	(47%)	20	(77%)
Geographic Region						
Northeast	35	(23%)	15	(21%)	6	(23%)
South	53	(35%)	25	(36%)	10	(38%)
Midwest	40	(26%)	19	(27%)	6	(23%)
West	24	(16%)	7	(12%)	4	(15%)
Within a MSA	135	(86%)	60	(86%)	22	(85%)
NIH Funding						
Top Tercile	40	(26%)	17	(24%)	5	(19%)
Middle Tercile	41	(27%)	20	(29%)	11	(42%)
Bottom Tercile	43	(28%)	20	(29%)	7	(27%)
None	28	(18%)	13	(19%)	3	(12%)

EBM is the topic of its own pre-clinical class at six of the schools reviewed. Six additional schools have a pre-clinical epidemiology and biostatistics class that includes EBM topics. At eight schools, EBM is a topic taught within one of the other pre-clinical courses.

At all schools, training in and practice of EBM is listed as an objective in one or more of the clinical clerkships. An EBM project is a required assignment in at least one of the clerkships at nine of the schools. Most commonly, the students identify a clinical question from one of their patient care experiences and search the literature to answer that question, writing a report and/or making a presentation to their peers. Six schools also have EBM as a topic in one of the classroom-based courses in the clinical years.

Quality Improvement Methods. We found an introduction to the concept of quality or quality improvement methods mentioned as an objective or a topic of specific instruction in 11 schools. At one school, there is a one-week mini-course on health care improvement in the third year, between rotations. In two schools all students participate in a Continuous Quality Improvement (CQI) project, and at a third school the students have the option of doing a CQI or EBM project.

Using Decision Aids. The curricula of three schools list using critical pathways and clinical practice guidelines as an objective in the internal medicine clerkships. Other decisions aids are not mentioned in any of the other curricula reviewed.

Systems-Based Practice

In the curricula of four schools, there is an indication of instruction in the general concepts in systems-based care. At one school, in a classroom-based course placed in the clerkship years, there are lectures in systems thinking and theory. Another school has similar instruction, with leadership skills and organizational theories in a preclinical class. In a third program, students complete a systems-based practice paper (e.g., comparing health plans or systems, describing a system-improvement project, and discussing health care system effects on access to care) while on an ambulatory medicine clerkship. Finally, at one school, there is a specific rotation during which students follow patients from hospital admission through discharge to obtain a broad view of the system of care, including issues relevant to quality, safety, and transitions for an individual patient.

Patient Care Coordination. Learning the principles of patient care coordination is often a core objective in clerkship experiences. At 12 schools, learning about coordination of care in the outpatient setting is an objective of a family medicine or ambulatory care clerkship. At five schools, coordination between inpatient providers is listed as an objective in the IM clerkship; however, often this is in relationship to coordinating between inpatient consultation services rather than provider hand-offs. Finally, seven schools list coordination of care at discharge as a skill to be learned, ranging from generating the discharge summary to coordinating post-discharge home services. One school has all IM clerkship students complete a post-discharge follow up phone call.

Working in Multidisciplinary Teams. Ten of the schools have working in multidisciplinary teams, or learning how to collaborate with non- physician health professionals, as an objective of the clinical rotations. Three schools additionally introduce this concept in a pre- clinical course.

Awareness of Health Care Costs and Financing. Awareness of health care costs is included in, or an objective of, at least one reviewed course curricula in 15 of the schools. Among these, the emphasis in the curricula on health care costs varies widely; three schools list this topic in all the reviewed curricula, while eight schools list it just once. At two of the schools, the students engage in simulated patient exercises, in which students are provided with and have to consider cost and insurance information in their diagnostic and treatment plans.

Interpersonal and Communication Skills

In all the curricula reviewed, a significant emphasis is placed on the basics of physician interpersonal and communication skills. These skills are commonly introduced in the pre-clinical years and then practiced and built on in clinical rotations.

Communicating with other Health Care Providers. Basic skills for communicating with other health care providers, such as writing notes and making oral presentations, are commonly taught in a pre-clinical class that simultaneously teach students techniques of patient interviewing and physical exams. Although schools have different names and formats for these courses, common names are "Clinical Skills" and "Introduction to Clinical Medicine." These skills are practiced and further developed in the pre-clinical preceptorships and clinical rotations. In all the schools, clinical rotations list the ability to function and communicate with the health care team as a key objective. During these rotations, students practice and receive feedback on writing notes, making informal and formal presentations of patient data, and, under the supervision of residents and faculty, discussing patient care with consultants.

Communicating with Patients. Among all schools reviewed, the basics of patient communication skills are introduced in a pre-clinical "Clinical Skills" class. The focus of this instruction is in eliciting a medical history from the patient. Other advanced topics, such as shared decisionmaking, patient education, and motivational interviewing, are addressed in these pre-clinical courses at nine schools.

Advanced communication skills are more commonly listed as objectives in clinical rotations. Shared decisionmaking skills are listed as a key objective or competency in at least one clinical rotation at 12 schools. The skills of providing patient education are listed in one or more clinical rotations at 13 schools and counseling patients in adherence or behavior change is listed in nine schools.

All of the medical schools use standardized patients for teaching and evaluating interpersonal and communication skills. Standardized patients are actors trained to provide the patient with pre-determined interview responses, sometime presenting a communication challenge. The student is observed by a faculty member (in person, or by video), who assesses the student's clinical skills, including communication. The standardized patient may also rate the students' communication skills.

Communicating with Special Populations. The curricula of all schools indicate training in cultural competency. In 18 schools, topics relevant to cultural competency, diversity, and/or racial issues in medicine are introduced during their clinical skills course or a parallel course. This is done through lectures, videos, readings, and, in a few schools, having community members speak on their perspectives on racial issues in the practice of medicine. The curricula of six schools contain instruction in using interpreters and four have a specific mention of working with patients with limited health literacy.

Communicating about End-of-Life Issues and Advanced Directives

In 23 of the 26 schools, communicating about end-of-life issues is included in the written curricula. The extent and approach to this education varies. Some schools have it listed as an objective of clerkships, without further detail. However, lectures, videos, and small-group discussions are also used in pre-clinical courses and classroom-based courses in the clinical years. One school has a two- week classroom course (between clerkships) that specifically addresses end-of-life issues and includes instruction on pain and palliative care topics, an orientation to pastoral care, and multicultural issues at the end of life.

Care Settings and Information Technology (IT) Infrastructure

Diverse Care Settings. Students at all schools have some clinical experiences outside the academic center; the quantity and nature of these experiences varies between schools. In 17 schools, students are initially introduced to community-based practices in a required preceptorship experiences in the preclinical years. At one school, this preceptorship site acts as a continuity clinic; the student continues going to the same clinic throughout the first three years and can elect to continue it in the fourth year.

In 12 schools, all students are assigned to a community site for their ambulatory medicine and/or family medicine rotation. In the remaining 14 schools, some students, but not all, will have a community- based ambulatory medicine or family practice placement.

Exposure to rural medicine is an explicit part of the curricula at a few of the schools. One school requires all students to do a two- month preceptorship in a rural community practice between the first and second year of instruction, with the explicit goal of observing the practice of medicine in the community. Another school has an extended interdisciplinary rural medicine block as part of its third year curriculum. Some other schools have a four-week rotation in the fourth year in which students can elect to be placed in an urban or rural community practice.

As part of the ambulatory medicine and geriatrics clerkship, two schools require experiences in private community faculty offices, nursing homes, rehabilitation clinics, hospice, and home care agencies. Two additional schools require home visits as part of this clerkship. One school requires a clerkship in rehabilitation medicine.

Some schools require students to experience non-clinical community settings or activities. Examples include participating in an Alcoholics Anonymous (AA) meetings, homeless shelters, and community health fairs.

Electronic Medical Record (EMR) & Computer Order Entry (COE). The curricula of four schools listed the appropriate use of EMR as a key objective in its clinical rotations. For the remainder of the schools, the syllabi did not mention the EMR or only indicated that orientation to the hospital or clinic system is provided. We could not discern from curricula the features of the EMR(s) that students are using in clinical experiences.

Discussion

Of the topics of interest, those most consistently appearing in the curricula of the reviewed medical schools are instruction in EBM, the basics of communication skills, cultural competency, and communicating about end-of-life issues. The first three of these topics are explicitly stated as standards in accreditation by The Liaison Committee on Medical Education (LCME).[37]

Schools appear, from their written curricula, to be highly varied in the inclusion of other topics. At several schools, one particular topic is highly emphasized and developed. For example, at a few schools, the provision of cost-effective care is integral to all curricula reviewed. At other schools, curricula in systems-based care, quality, and end-of-life issues are emphasized. As in the IM residency programs that were interviewed in this study, the focus on these topics may reflect the interests and expertise of the institution's faculty. Other institutional or community factors may also be acting as facilitators and/or barriers to innovation in developing the curricula in these topics. Exploring the etiologies behind these differences would inform policies to encourage inclusion of these topics.

Limitations

The written curricula also vary in detail and quality, which is a limitation of this assessment. Furthermore, this assessment is based on written objectives for courses, without assessment of the implementation or effectiveness of the implemented curricula. For example, although the written objectives of a clerkship may include students learning and practicing the delivery of evidence-based, culturally sensitive, cost- effective, and patient-centered care, the extent to which these curricular elements are implemented may be incomplete or ineffective. Similarly, faculty may be consistently teaching these topics during patient care, even though they are not written explicitly into the curricula. Assessing the competency of medical students in these topics would be needed to get the most accurate measure of medical school teaching.

Another limitation of this data is in the limited response rate of the medical schools; the schools that responded to our request may not be representative of the total population of U.S. medical schools. Further, this sample is limited to U.S. medical schools and thus is not a reflection of the education of international medical school graduates (IMGs). Given that 26 percent of all residents graduate from non-U.S. medical schools[37] and, as several IM program directors noted, that the undergraduate medical education of IMGs may be quite different in the topics of interest, there is a need to understand IMG knowledge and skill in these topics.

Next Steps

This exploratory analysis of medical school written curricula shows some areas of commonality, but also much variability, in the emphasis given to the topics of interest. The next steps would be to explore whether this variability is also present in the implemented curricula, the factors that have led to actual variability, and the characteristics of the programs that have been most successful in developing skills and knowledge in practice-based learning and improvement; systems-based care; interpersonal and communication skills.

Appendix B: Interview Protocol

Preparing Physicians for 21st Century Challenges- Interview Protocol –IM Programs

Introduction

In this interview, we will be asking about your program's training in engaging in practice-based learning and improvement, system-based practice, and interpersonal and communication skills. We will be asking individual topics within each domain, asking if your program provides training in these topics, for details on that training, and then how well you think your program prepares your residents in these areas. At the end of each section, we will additionally ask about enablers, barriers and facilitators that you and/or your program have experienced in approaching training in these topics. We will end with giving you the opportunity to comment in general with about enablers, barriers and facilitators to innovation in graduate medical education.

RAND will not disclose your identity or specific information that identifies you to anyone outside of the research team. We will destroy all information that identifies you at the end of the study. The risks to you by participating to you are minimal. However, there is a small professional risk to you by expressing your impressions and opinion of your program's curriculum. To minimize this risk, we will be safeguarding your identify and the identity of your institution. You do not have to participate and can decline to answer any question or stop the interview for any reason at any time.

Do you have any questions? Is it ok to proceed?

Before beginning, I would also like to ask for permission to record this interview. This recording will only be used to ensure that our notes are accurate and the recording will be accessible only to study personnel, without identifying information, and will be destroyed at the end of the study. If you would like us to turn off the recording at any point you can just let us know. Is it ok if we begin recording?

Practice-Based Learning and Improvement

In this first section, we would like to ask you about your program's training in engaging in practice-based learning and improvement.

Of note, we define training as both the formal elements–lectures, conferences, projects, etc , and informal training, through clinical experiences or interactions with faculty, staff and patients.

	(a) Does your program train its residents in	(b) (If yes) Can you describe your program's training in this subject? (specific probes to be used if not spontaneously mentioned)	(c) (If Yes) In preparing your residents for their practice after they finish training, do you believe that the preparation your program provides in this subject is_______				
First I would like to ask about your training in Quality Improvement Methods. We have broken this training into its two component parts - 1) Systematically analyzing the quality of care being provided in one's own or a group's practice and 2) Implementing system changes with the goal of practice improvement							
Systematically analyzing the quality of care being provided in one's own or a group's practice	□ Yes □ No	(Disease registries? Lectures? Project? – Individual or Small group?)	Excellent	Very Good	Good	Fair	Poor
Implementing system changes with the goal of practice improvement	□ Yes □ No	(Lectures? Project? – Some or all residents)	Excellent	Very Good	Good	Fair	Poor
Now I am going to ask about how you teach evidence-based medicine							
Searching scientific literature to answer questions	□ Yes □ No	(Lectures?)	Excellent	Very Good	Good	Fair	Poor
Critiquing medical literature and applying it to clinical decisions	□ Yes □ No	(Lectures? Journal Club?)	Excellent	Very Good	Good	Fair	Poor

(Continued)

Using electronic medical records	□ Yes □ No	(At all sites, some sites, no sites Inpatient v. Outpatient)	Excellent	Very Good	Good	Fair	Poor
Using computer-order entry	□ Yes □ No	(At all sites, some sites, no sites Inpatient v. Outpatient)	Excellent	Very Good	Good	Fair	Poor
Using clinical prediction rules or decision-aids to guide care	□ Yes □ No	(Clinical Pathways, Ordersets, rediction Rules IT supported?)	Excellent	Very Good	Good	Fair	Poor

Are there other areas in which your program trains residents in practice-based learning? □ No □ Yes (please specify)

In the areas of practice-based learning and improvement that you indicated your training to be excellent or very good (remind respondent of these areas), what have been key resources or factors that have facilitated your program's ability to provide this training? (probe for details as needed)

Systems-Based Practice

In this section, we would like to ask you about your program's training in engaging in system-based practice.

Again, we define training as both the formal elements– lectures, conferences, projects, etc , and informal training, through clinical experiences or interactions with faculty, staff and patients.

	Does your program train its residents in	(If yes) Can you describe your program's training in this subject?	(If Yes) Presently, in preparing your trainees for their post-residency practices, do you believe the training your program provides in this subject is___________				
Using methods for improving patient safety	□ Yes □ No	Lectures/Projects Lectures on theories, methods?	Excellent	Very Good	Good	Fair	Poor
In the next 3 questions, I'd like to ask about how your program trains its resident to communicate and coordinate patient care across 3 different types of transitions – first, across provider hand-offs in the hospital, secondly at the time of hospital discharge, and thirdly, for patients in the outpatient setting, who have not been hospitalized but have multiple providers.							
Communicating & coordinating patient care across provider hand-offs in the hospital	□ Yes □ No	Lectures ? IT based?	Excellent	Very Good	Good	Fair	Poor
Communicating & coordinating patient care at hospital discharge	□ Yes □ No	Lectures ? IT based?	Excellent	Very Good	Good	Fair	Poor
Communicating & coordinating patient care among multiple providers in outpatient settings	□ Yes □ No	Lectures ? IT based?	Excellent	Very Good	Good	Fair	Poor
Working in multidisciplinary teams	□ Yes □ No	(Inpatient – round together, scheduled meetings? Outpatient - Scheduled Meetings or Projects?)	Excellent	Very Good	Good	Fair	Poor
Working in managed care settings	□ Yes □ No	(Lectures/ Didactics Experience)	Excellent	Very Good	Good	Fair	Poor
Working in "medical homes"	□ Yes □ No		Excellent	Very Good	Good	Fair	Poor
Knowing absolute or relative costs of various treatments & diagnostic tests	□ Yes □ No	(Lectures?)	Excellent	Very Good	Good	Fair	Poor
Knowing how much patients have to pay out-of-pocket for various treatments & diagnostic tests	□ Yes □ No	(Lectures?)	Excellent	Very Good	Good	Fair	Poor
Now I would like to ask about the different settings in which your residents gain experience. Do your residents have any required experiences in: A Community Clinic or Private Practitioner's Office? □ Yes □ No Providing Hospice or Palliative Care? □ Yes □ No Conducting Home Visits? □ Yes □ No Nursing Homes or Rehabilitation Units? □ Yes □ No							

Are there other areas in which your program trains residents in systems-based practice? □ No □ Yes (please specify)

In the areas of systems-based practice that you have indicated your training to be excellent or very good (remind respondent of these areas), what have been key resources or factors that have facilitated your program's ability to provide this training? (probe for details as needed)

Section 4 - Interpersonal and Communication Skills

In this section, we would like to ask you about your program's training in interpersonal and communication skills.

Again, for each section we define training as both the formal elements– lectures, conferences, projects, etc , and informal training, through clinical experiences or interactions with faculty, staff and patients.

	Does your program train its residents in	(If yes) Can you describe your program's training in this subject?	(If Yes) Presently, in preparing your trainees for their postresidency practices, do you believe the training your program provides in this subject is__________				
Communicating with other healthcare providers (physicians and non-physicians)	□ Yes □ No	(Lectures or other specific training?)	Excellent	Very Good	Good	Fair	Poor
Communicating clearly with patients about diagnosis and treatment plans	□ Yes □ No	(Lectures or other specific training?)	Excellent	Very Good	Good	Fair	Poor
Engaging patients in shared decision-making	□ Yes □ No	(Lectures or other specific training?)	Excellent	Very Good	Good	Fair	Poor
Providing patient education about self-care activities	□ Yes □ No	(Lectures/ training on how to do patient education?IT resources?)	Excellent	Very Good	Good	Fair	Poor

(Continued)

Provide counseling to enhance adherence or behavior change	□ Yes □ No	(Lectures or other specific training?)	Excellent	Very Good	Good	Fair	Poor
Communicating with patients with low health literacy	□ Yes □ No	(Lectures or other specific training?)	Excellent	Very Good	Good	Fair	Poor
Acquiring cultural-competency	□ Yes □ No	(Lectures or other specific training?)	Excellent	Very Good	Good	Fair	Poor
Working with interpreters	□ Yes □ No	(Lectures or other specific training?)	Excellent	Very Good	Good	Fair	Poor
Communicating with patients about end-of-life decisions or palliative care	□ Yes □ No	(Lectures or other specific training? Teaching in advanced directives?)	Excellent	Very Good	Good	Fair	Poor
Communicating with the patients' family and significant others such as holding family meetings	□ Yes □ No	(Lectures or other specific training?)	Excellent	Very Good	Good	Fair	Poor

Are there other areas in which your program trains residents in interpersonal and communication skills? □ No □ Yes (please specify)

In the areas of interpersonal and communication skills that you have indicated your training to be excellent or very good (remind respondent of these areas), what have been key resources or factors that have facilitated your program's ability to provide this training? (probe for details as needed)

Section 5- Conclusion

I would like to end with asking if you think there are other general enablers and facilitators or barriers to innovation in graduate medical education that you have not already mentioned?

Finally, are there any topics of questions that were not covered in this interview that you think should be or would like to comment upon?

Thank you very much for your time. This information is very helpful. Although I believe we have everything we need, if we have any details that need clarification, would it be ok for us to contact you again?

Yes No

Thank you again and have a nice day.

REFERENCES

[1] U.S. Census Bureau. Minority Population Tops 100 Million. Available at: http://www.census.gov/PressRelease/www/releases/archives/ pop ulation/010048 .html. Accessed August 15, 2008.

[2] National Center for Health Statistics. Trends In Health and Aging. *Centers for Disease Control.* Available at: http://www.cdc.go v/nchs/agingact.htm. Accessed August 15. 2008.

[3] Wolff, JL; Starfield, B; Anderson, G. Prevalence, Expenditures, and Complications of Multiple Chronic Conditions in the Elderly. *Arch Intern Med*, 2002, 162, 2269-2276.

[4] Institute of Medicine. Health Professions Education: *A Bridge to Quality*. Washington, DC: The National Academies Press; 2003.

[5] Council on Graduate Medical Education. *Physician Education for a Changing Health Care Environment*. Washington, DC: Health Resources and Services Administration; 1999.

[6] Institute of Medicine. Crossing the Quality Chasm. Washington, DC: The National Academies Press; 2001.

[7] Association of American Medical Colleges. Learning Objectives for Medical Student Education: *Guidelines for Medical Schools*. Available at: http://www.aamc.org/meded/msop/. Accessed August 19, 2008.

[8] The Pew Health Professions Commission. Health professions education and managed care: Challenges and necessary responses. *Report on the*

Advisory Panel on Health Professions Education and Managed Care, 1995.
[9] Blumenthal, D. Training Tomorrow's Doctors: The Medical Education Mission of Academic Health Centers. New York, NY: *The Commonwealth Fund*, 2002.
[10] Commission On Osteopathic College Accreditation. Accreditation of Colleges Of Osteopathic Medicine: COM Accreditation Standards and Procedures. Available at: http://www.osteopathic.org/index.cfm?PageID=acc_predoc. Accessed August 15, 2008.
[11] Accreditation Council for Graduate Medical Education. Common Program Requirements. Available at http://www.acgme.org/acWebsite /dutyHours/dh_dutyhoursCommonPR070 12007.pdf. Accessed January 7th, 2009
[12] McGlynn, EA. et al., !The Quality of Health Care Delivered to Adults in the United States,! *New England Journal of Medicine*, 348, no. 26 (2003), 2635-2645.
[13] ACGME. Common Program Requirements. Available at http://www.acgme.org/acWebsite/dutyHours/dh_dutyhoursCommonPR0 70 12007.pdf, accessed January 4th, 2009.
[14] Wolff, JL; Starfield, B; Anderson, G. Prevalence, Expenditures, and Complications of Multiple Chronic Conditions in the Elderly. *Arch Intern Med*, 2002,162, 2269-2276.
[15] Shortell, SM; Gillies, RR; Anderson, DA. Remaking Health Care in America. 2nd ed. San Francisco, CA: Jossey-Bass; 2000.
[16] Shine KI. Health care quality and how to achieve it. *Acad Med*, 2002, 77, 91-99.
[17] Lorig, KR; Sobel, DS; Ritter, PL; et al. Effect of a self- management program on patients with chronic disease. *Eff Clin Pract*, 2001, 4(6), 256-262.
[18] Institute of Medicine. *A Prescription To End Confusion*. Washington, DC: The National Academies Press; 2004.
[19] Pérez-Stable, EJ; Nápoles-Springer, A; Miramontes, JM. The Effects of Ethnicity and Language on Medical Outcomes of Patients with Hypertension or Diabetes. *Med Care*, 1997, 35 (12), 1212-1219.
[20] Betancourt, JR; Green, AR; Carrillo, JE; Park, ER. Cultural Competence And Health Care Disparities: Key Perspectives And Trends. *Health Aff*, 2005, 24(2), 499-505.

[21] Association of American Medical Colleges. Cultural Competence Education. Available at: http://www.aamc.org/meded/tacct/culturalcomped.pdf. Accessed August 15, 2008.

[22] Institute of Medicine. *Unequal Treatment. Washington*, DC: The National Academies Press; 2001.

[23] Gorman, PJ; Meier, AH; Rawn, C; Krummel, TM. The future of medical education is no longer blood and guts, it is bits and bytes. *Am J Surg.*, 2000, 180(5), 353-356.

[24] Hunt, DL; Haynes, RB; Hanna, SE; Smith, K. Effects of Computer-Based Clinical Decision Support Systems on Physician Performance and Patient Outcomes: *A Systematic Review JAMA*, 1998, 280(15), 1339-1346.

[25] Dexter, PR; Perfkins, S; Overhage, JM; et al. A Computerized Reminder System To Increase the Use of Preventive Care for Hospitalized Patients. *N Engl J Med*, 2001, 345(13), 965-970.

[26] American College of Physicians http://www.acponline.org/medical Accessed September 22nd, 2008.

[27] Accreditation Council for Graduate Medical Education. Common Program Requirements. Available at http://www.acgme.org/acWebsite/dutyHours/dh_dutyhoursCommonPR070 12007.pdf. Accessed January 7th, 2009.

[28] American Medical Association (AMA) Fellowship and Residency Electronic Interactive Database (FREIDA). Available at http://www.ama assn.org/ama/pub/category/2997.html. Accessed November 24th, 2008.

[29] The American Board of Internal Medicine. Practice Improvement Modules. Available at: http://www.abim.org/pims/default.aspx. Accessed January 5th, 2009.

[30] The Kenneth B. Schwartz Center. Available at: http://www.theschwartzcenter.org/programs/rounds.html. Accessed December 28th, 2008.

[31] The Institute of Medicine. Resident Duty Hours: Enhancing Sleep, Supervision, and Safety. Washington, DC: The National Academies Press; 2008.

[32] Wynn, B; Guarino, C; Morse, L; Cho, M. Alternative Ways of Financing Graduate Medical Education. Available at: http://aspe.hhs.gov/health df. Accessed January 12, 2009.

[33] http://www.lcme.org/directry.htm and http:// www. osteopathic. org/index. cfm?PageID=sir_college

[34] http://www.census.gov/geo/www/us_regdiv.pdf

[35] Terciles calculated from dollar amounts reported at: http://report.nih.gov/award/trends/FindOrg.cfm
[36] Association of American Medical Colleges. Curriculum Directory. Available at: http://services.Accessed Sep-tember 25th, 2008.
[37] Liason Committee on Graduate Medical Education. Current Standards. Available at: http://www.lcme.org/functionslist.htm#educational% 20 program, accessed January 9th, 2009.
[38] The American Medical Association. International Medical Graduates in the U.S. Workforce. Available at: http://www.ama-assn.org/ama1/pub/upload/mm/18/img-workforcepaper.pdf, accessed January 3rd, 2009.

End Notes

[1] MedPAC originally requested that RAND conduct a two-part study: 1) assessing the written curricula of IM programs and 2) conducting semi-structured interviews with IM program directors. However, despite sending requests to 70 programs, we were able to obtain complete written curricula from only 8 programs. Reasons for refusal included: (1) Not having the time to compile the numerous curricula components; (2) Concerns about maintaining intellectual property rights; (3) Current written curricula being out-of-date or under revision. Due to the inadequate response, MedPAC and RAND jointly decided to discontinue the assessment of written curricula.

[2] MedPAC requested RAND conduct at least 25 interviews. RAND predetermined that the minimum acceptable response rate would be 40%. We initially sent requests to 60 programs to achieve the minimum response rate with 25 responses. One of the 60 programs was later determined to be ineligible as it did not graduate residents in 2008. Therefore, our requests were sent to 59 eligible programs.

[3] At the time of the interview, we asked if the director had received our email with the interview information, provided them an opportunity to ask questions, and then requested their verbal consent to proceed with the interview. If the director did not recall receiving the information email, we read the information to them before requesting consent. The Human Subjects Committee of the RAND Corporation approved the study protocol.

[4] We additionally asked directors to rate their programs teaching on these topics, in relation to the preparation needed for residents' post-training practices. However, directors appeared to have wide variation in their perceptions of the preparation needed in each of these topics, which limited the validity of this data. Thus, the results of these ratings are not presented in this report.

[5] Under certain circumstances, patient care activities in non- hospital associated ambulatory settings are reimbursed; however, the associated rules and requirements are prohibitive in their complexity. This issue is beyond the scope of this study and was not specifically discussed with the directors, except that several directors volunteered their impressions that rotating their residents into these setting was not a financially – viable option.

In: Graduate Medical Education Issues
Editor: Caroline I. Hansen et al.
ISBN: 978-1-61122-902-8

Chapter 2

MEDICAL EDUCATION IN THE UNITED STATES: SUPPORTING LONG-TERM DELIVERY SYSTEM REFORMS

MedPac

SUMMARY

Spending an estimated $9 billion in 2008, Medicare is the largest financial supporter of graduate medical education. Averaging almost $100,000 per resident per year, Medicare subsidizes education and training for about 90,000 residents in more than 1,100 hospitals through direct and indirect payments for graduate medical education. To some extent, this federal support signals the societal value the Congress places on educating and training our physicians. Despite this spending, however, a number of reports and articles have expressed concern that our health professionals are not gaining certain skills they need to provide the kinds of care that will best serve the public's needs.

Reforming medical education will be a key component in transforming the nation's health care delivery system from one that historically has focused on care for acute illness—at the expense of chronic condition management, coordination of care across settings, and disease prevention—to one that values patient-centered care, quality improvement, and resource conservation. Our medical schools and residency programs need to emphasize a set of skills and knowledge that will equip students and residents to practice and lead in reformed delivery systems that work under restructured payment incentives.

In considering ways to reform both health care delivery and medical education and training in the United States, this chapter offers an initial focus on physicians. Specifically, it reviews the multifaceted process of becoming a practicing physician, including the organizations involved in accreditation and certification; the costs and benefits for hospitals and physicians involved in teaching and supervising residents; internal medicine residency programs' curricula as they relate to health delivery system reforms; and the financial disincentives and regulatory issues that discourage residency rotations in nonhospital settings.

Residency programs' curricula are not well aligned with objectives of delivery system reform—To learn about how selected curricula are presented in residency programs, we contracted with RAND researchers to conduct a series of semistructured interviews with directors from 26 internal medicine residency programs. This study found that, although most programs provide at least some formal instruction in selected topics essential for delivery reform (e.g., care coordination across settings), overall their curricula fall far short of instruction recommended by the Institute of Medicine and other experts (Cordasco et al. 2009). Of particular concern is the relative lack of formal instruction and experience in multidisciplinary teamwork, cost awareness in clinical decision making, comprehensive health information technology, and patient care in ambulatory settings. Reform-related topics that were reported to be covered more consistently in residency programs are evidence-based medicine and communicating with patients about end-of-life care. As may be expected, researchers found large variations in the extent of and approach to teaching, and program directors reported multiple factors that facilitate or impede their ability to instruct in topics related to delivery system reform. Faculty expertise in selected topics, such as quality measurement, can strongly influence residents' skills and experience.

Financial incentives and regulatory issues discourage nonhospital residency experience—Residency programs are largely based in teaching hospitals. These hospitals face financial and regulatory incentives to keep residents in the hospital for their education and training rather than encourage them to rotate to nonhospital settings. Consequently, residents spend most of their time involved in caring for acutely ill hospital inpatients. This hospital-based experience provides residents with important skills for treating serious illnesses, but it must be balanced with sufficient education and training in nonhospital and community-based settings. Devoting too much resident time in the hospital setting can be problematic, as most of the medical conditions that practicing physicians confront are, and should be, managed in nonhospital settings (e.g., physician offices, nursing facilities, and patient homes). The development of skills in these nonhospital settings is important for patient health, patient comfort, and health care spending.

While accreditation organizations specifically require ambulatory experience for many specialties, Medicare places no requirements on residency programs. Many programs satisfy their accreditation requirements for ambulatory care through residency rotations in hospital outpatient departments, rather than nonhospital settings. The reluctance of teaching hospitals to have residents rotate outside the hospital can be attributed to historical patterns of medical education, regulatory issues, and financial incentives. For example, under current statute and regulations, in certain circumstances, when residents rotate to nonhospital settings, teaching hospitals may lose some of the funding they could otherwise receive through Medicare's graduate medical education payments. Hospitals face an even greater financial incentive to keep residents within the hospital to retain the clinical labor that residents provide.

Future issues for exploration—Future Commission work will stem not only from the findings of work presented in this chapter but also from exploring other issues and questions on the topic of medical education in the United States. Thus, in addition to analyzing specific ways to encourage more residency experience in nonhospital settings, further analysis will focus on three main areas:

- *Linking delivery system reforms to medical education incentives*—The Commission recognizes that residents and other health care professionals will best learn the skills needed to provide high-quality, efficient care when medical education occurs in settings where such care is actually performed. Thus, the Commission will explore policies that might link medical education incentives with delivery system reforms.
- *Structuring medical education subsidies to produce the professionals we need*—Among physicians, nurses, and physician assistants, medical education incentives could be helpful in achieving the optimal balance of generalists and specialists to help reform our

health care delivery system. The Commission will examine possible ways to address this issue as well as ways to increase the diversity of medical school enrollment.

- *Enlisting other payers to contribute explicitly to medical education*—Considering the shared societal benefits of high-quality medical education for patients of all ages, the Commission will analyze options that expand contributions from other health care payers for medical education. This analysis also could explore potential mechanisms for distributing collected funds equitably and efficiently across settings and programs.

Spending an estimated $9 billion in 2008, Medicare is the largest financial supporter of graduate medical education. Averaging almost $100,000 per resident per year, Medicare subsidizes education and training for about 90,000 residents in more than 1,100 hospitals through direct and indirect payments for graduate medical education. To some extent, this federal support signals the societal value the Congress places on educating and training physicians. Despite this spending, however, a number of reports and articles have expressed concern that our health professionals are not gaining certain skills they need to perform the kinds of care that will best serve the public's needs (Blue Ridge Academic Health Group 2003, Blumenthal 2002, COGME 2007, Holmboe et al. 2005, IOM 2008, IOM 2003, Ludmerer and Johns 2005, Meyers et al. 2007, Mullan 2009, Weinberger et al. 2006).

Reforming medical education will be a key component in transforming the nation's health care delivery system from one that historically has focused on care for acute illness—at the expense of chronic condition management, coordination of care across settings, and disease prevention—to one that values patient-centered care, quality improvement, and resource conservation. Our medical schools and residency programs need to emphasize a set of skills and knowledge that will equip students and residents to practice and lead in reformed delivery systems that work under restructured payment incentives.

In considering ways to reform both health care delivery and medical education and training in the United States, this chapter offers an initial focus on physicians. In addition to background information on physician education, we examine the federal funding policies that bias medical education heavily toward acute hospital care.

PROCESS OF BECOMING A PHYSICIAN AND CONTINUING PRACTICE

The process of becoming a practicing physician is multifaceted. It starts with undergraduate preparation, followed by four years of medical school, a minimum of three years of graduate medical education in a specialty, and potentially further instruction in a subspecialty. Physicians must also obtain a medical license in order to practice independently. After completing a residency program, physicians may—and most do—seek specialty board certification. Throughout their years of practice, physicians maintain their medical license through continuing medical education (CME). They also maintain their board certification by fulfilling a comprehensive, multifaceted mix of requirements over a set period of time (Figure 1-1, p. 8).

Undergraduate Preparation

The journey to becoming a physician begins at the undergraduate level, where students must fulfill basic premed coursework requirements (biology, chemistry, mathematics, physics, and English), while maintaining a well-rounded undergraduate experience that includes coursework in humanities and social sciences. Medical schools also look favorably on applicants who volunteer at local hospitals and clinics (AAMC 2009). The average student applies for admission to 13 allopathic medical schools. For the 2007–2008 academic year, more than 42,000 people applied for a little more than 18,000 first- year positions (AAMC 2008a).[1] Almost all medical schools require students to take the Medical College Admission Test, which is a standardized, multiple-choice examination designed to assess students' problem-solving ability, critical thinking, writing skills, and knowledge of science concepts and principles prerequisite to the study of medicine.

Medical School

Medical school usually lasts four years. Each medical school differs in how it organizes its program. In general, during the first two years, students study the sciences basic to medicine: anatomy, biochemistry, physiology, microbiology, pathology, pharmacology, and behavioral sciences. In addition, they are introduced to basic interviewing and examination techniques. In the third year, students start clinical clerkships, where they gain clinical experience in hospitals and other settings. These third-year clerkships are usually in internal medicine, family medicine, pediatrics, obstetrics and gynecology, general surgery, and psychiatry. In the fourth year clinical rotations continue, although students often focus on specific subfields.

During the fourth year of medical school, students decide on the specialty they want to pursue and participate in the National Residency Matching Program (NRMP), a matching service that uses a computer algorithm to match applicants to programs according to the preferences of the medical students and residency programs.[2] Through the NRMP, students can choose from 26 core specialties. Virtually all medical students participate in the match to be assigned to a residency program. Only after the matchis complete can students who are not successfully matched attempt to pursue slots left unfilled by the matching process. A match between an applicant and a program is considered a binding commitment.[3]

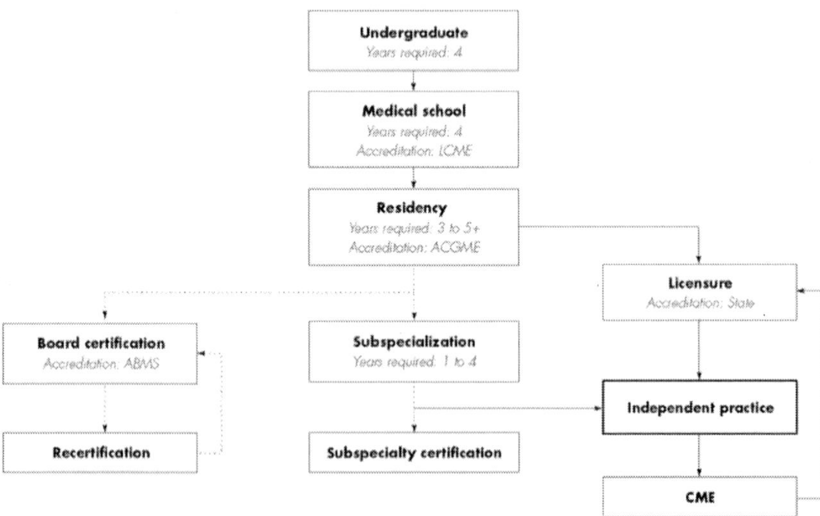

Note: LCME (Liaison Committee on Medical Education), ACGME (Accreditation Council for Graduate Medical Education), ABMS (American Board of Medical Specialties), CME (continuing medical education). Solid flow lines indicate required paths. Dotted flow lines indicate optional paths. Most physicians seek board certification. Physicians may seek subspecialization after completion of their residency.

Figure 1-1. The process of becoming a physician and continuing practice

Diversity in Medical Education

Medical students tend to come from relatively affluent families. In 2005, 55 percent of students came from families in the top quintile of family income; only about 5 percent came from families in the lowest quintile (Figure 1-2) (AAMC 2008b). This trend has been fairly consistent for the past 20 years. Given the association of college graduation with family income, some skewing can be expected in medical school enrollment toward higher income families; nevertheless, the U.S. medical school enrollment figures show an overwhelming lack of economic diversity among students and subsequently among practicing physicians entering the profession.

The racial and ethnic composition of medical school enrollees also is not representative of the population at large (Table 1-1). For instance, for the 2007–2008 academic year, African Americans account for 12.3 percent of the U.S. population, but just 6.3 percent of allopathic and 3.5 percent of osteopathic medical school matriculants (first-year enrollees). Similarly, Hispanics account for 15.1 percent of the U.S. population but just 7.9 percent of allopathic and 3.6 percent of osteopathic medical school matriculants. Asian Americans, on the other hand, make up 4.4 percent of the U.S. population but account for 19.8 percent of allopathic and 17.1 percent of osteopathic medical school matriculants. As in the general population, whites make up the largest share of students entering medical school.

Table 1-1 also shows that the demographic composition of medical school enrollment roughly parallels the proportion of applications medical schools receive. This suggests that factors such as financial and educational barriers affect students' decisions to apply to medical school and ultimately shape the demographics of the physician workforce. Although college graduation is one factor influencing minority enrollment, the proportion of African Americans and Hispanics in medical school has not increased much over the past decade, despite substantial increases in the number of African Americans and Hispanic students graduating from four-year colleges, including increases relative to whites in the number graduating with majors in biological and biomedical sciences (Grumbach and Mendoza 2008). This growth presents an opportunity for developing strategies to increase diversity in medical school enrollment.

There are a number of benefits to having an ethnically diverse physician workforce, and the Commission is concerned about this issue. Research has shown that a racially and ethnically diverse health care workforce is associated with better access to and quality of care for disadvantaged populations, greater patient choice and satisfaction, and better educational experiences for students in health professions (HRSA 2006, IOM 2004a, Komaromy et al. 1996, Mertz and Grumbach 2001, Moy and Bartman 1995). Greater diversity in the health professions would likely lead to improved public health by increasing access to care for underserved populations and by increasing opportunities for minority patients to see practitioners with whom they share a common race, ethnicity, or language. Race, ethnicity, and language concordance, which are associated with better patient–practitioner relationships and communication, may increase patients' likelihood of receiving and accepting appropriate medical care (HRSA 2006). From an educational standpoint, an ethnically diverse student body has been associated with better performance across all ethnicities on intellectual and civic development (IOM 2004a). As the nation becomes increasingly diverse, a business case can also be made for a health care workforce that is culturally and linguistically diverse and attuned to the population being served (Grumbach and Mendoza 2008).

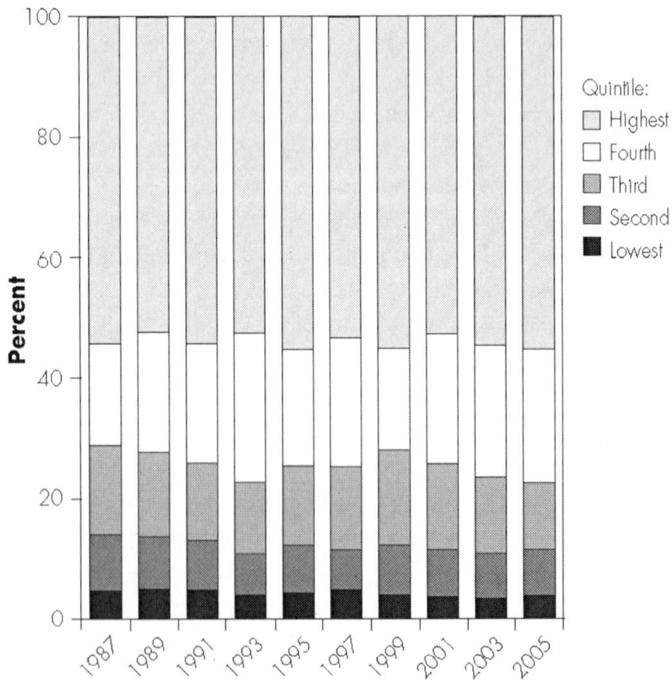

Source: Association of American Medical Colleges 2008.

Figure 1-2. Parent household income of entering medical students in U.S. medical schools, by quintiles, 1987–2005

Table 1-1. Racial and ethnic composition of medical school applicants and matriculants for the 2007–2008 academic year

Race/ ethnicity	U.S. population	Medical school			
		allopathic		Osteopathic	
		Applicants	Matriculants	Applicants	Matriculants
White	66.0%	56.4%	58.9%	59.4%	69.6%
Hispanic	15.1	7.3	7.9	6.4	3.6
Black or African American	12.3	7.2	6.3	5.9	3.5
Asian	4.4	19.6	19.8	19.5	17.1
Native American/ Alaskan native	0.9	0.3	0.3	0.6	0.8
Native Hawaiian/ Pacific Islander	0.1	0.3	0.2	0.1	*
Other/ unknown	1.2	9.0	6.5	8.2	5.4

Note: For the applicants and matriculants groups the "other/unknown" category includes foreign students who are not U.S. residents, individuals with more than one race, and individuals that did not provide their race. Totals may not sum to 100 percent due to rounding.

* Native Hawaiian and Pacific Islander included with Asian.

Source: Association of American Medical Colleges data warehouse applicant matriculant file as of October 10, 2008; American Association of Colleges of Osteopathic Medicine 2009 applicant and first-year enrollment data; and U.S. Census annual estimates of the population by sex, race, and Hispanic origin for the United States: April 1, 2000 to July 1, 2007.

Medical school students also appear to come disproportionately from urban areas, but research on this correlation is limited (Fordyce et al. 2007). Factors associated with lower rates of medical school enrollment among students from rural areas include lower income and less proximity to medical schools. Research suggests that medical students born in rural areas are more likely to select primary care specialties and to practice in rural areas (Brooks et al. 2002, Phillips et al. 2009). Therefore, geographic diversity among medical school students is important for maintaining access to care across the United States. In general, osteopathic medical schools enroll a proportionately higher share of rural students compared with allopathic medical schools (Peters et al. 1999).

Many decades ago women represented less than a quarter of U.S. medical school enrollees, but they now account for about half of all enrollees.

Student Debt

Although medical students are significantly more likely to come from higher income families, many graduate from medical school with sizable student debt from tuition and fees. Only 13 percent of medical students graduate without any educational debt. In 2008, the average student reported a debt load of $154,600, which is 11 percent higher than for the previous year. Today's graduates commit about 9 percent to 12 percent of their after-tax income for educational debt service (Steinbrook 2008). More than a quarter of graduates with indebtedness carried a debt of more than $200,000 (AAMC 2008c). Medical school students with higher debt are more likely to participate in loan repayment programs for underserved communities, such as the National Health Service Corps (Phillips et al. 2009). However, overall rates of U.S. medical school graduates practicing in these communities have fallen, particularly for primary care.

Graduate Medical Education

After completing medical school, graduates enter the residency programs to which they are assigned through the NRMP. During residency, residents gain more practical experience in a specific field of medicine. Most residency programs are sponsored by teaching hospitals or medical schools. Teaching hospitals are hospitals that participate in graduate medical education; a large proportion of residents' education takes place in inpatient and outpatient departments of teaching hospitals.

The length of time of residencies varies by specialty: from three years for the primary care specialties of family medicine, internal medicine, and pediatrics to five or more years for general surgery and other surgical specialties. Some specialties require a preliminary year of residency in internal medicine or general surgery before entering (e.g., dermatology, urology). When physicians graduate from a residency program, they are eligible to take their specialty board certification examinations. After completing a residency program, however, many new physicians subspecialize with additional fellowship years (e.g., cardiology, hand surgery), stretching the total length of education and training an additional one to four years, depending on the subspecialty.

Roughly one-quarter of all residents are graduates of medical schools located outside the United States and Canada. These international medical graduates (IMGs) must also be certified by the Educational Commission for Foreign Medical Graduates (ECFMG) before entering an approved residency. The ECFMG assesses the readiness of IMGs to enter residency programs accredited by the Accreditation Council for Graduate Medical Education (ACGME). A higher proportion of IMGs enter primary care residencies than other specialties (Salsberg et al. 2008).

Physician Licensure

States maintain their own rules for physicians' licensure. Licensure occurs through each state's medical licensing board and involves, among other requirements, passing the three-step United States Medical Licensing Examination (USMLE). The first two exams take place during medical school, and the third takes place during the first year of residency. To be licensed to practice independently, physicians must also complete a minimum number of years in an approved residency program, which varies by state and is typically one to two years. In most states and under most circumstances, physicians who graduate from an accredited medical school outside the United States or Canada or complete graduate medical education overseas are required to complete an ACGME-approved program before being licensed to practice medicine.

After they have completed their residencies and are licensed to practice, physicians maintain their competencies and licenses and learn about new and developing areas in medicine and their specialty by pursuing CME. Physicians may receive CME credits by attending approved lectures or conferences; reviewing certain publications; or using online programs, audio, video, or other electronic media designed to provide CME credits. All but five states require a minimum number of CME credits to maintain state licensure.[4] The number of CME credits required varies across jurisdictions; on average, states require 30 credit hours per year, with 11 states requiring as many as 50.[5] Some states mandate specific types of CME. California, for instance, requires all general internists and family physicians, for whom at least 20 percent of their patient population is 65 or older, to receive at least 20 percent of their CME hours in geriatric medicine or the care of older patients. Other states have requirements on HIV/AIDS care, risk management, and end-of-life palliative care (AMA 2008). In general, physicians are not required to get CME credits in areas related to their practice nor are they required to demonstrate to the state licensing boards what they have learned from CME activities (FSMB 2009).

Specialty Certification

After completing a residency, most physicians become board certified in their specialty. Specialty certification is voluntary and not required for state licensure. Many health plans and hospitals, however, require certification for inclusion in networks and hospital privileges. Specialty certification occurs through the medical specialty board for each specialty. To become eligible for board certification in a specialty, a physician must complete an approved residency in that specialty and have an institutional or valid license to practice medicine. A physician who meets these basic admission standards will be evaluated by a specialty board using written and oral examinations. Because specialties differ so widely, the criteria that inform these tests are quite different (ABMS 2009).

Most specialty boards require physicians to pass recertifying exams and meet other requirements to maintain their certification, also referred to as maintenance of certification (MOC). These other requirements include a minimum amount of CME relevant to their specialty and evidence of participation in practice-based assessment.[6] The time cycle for recertification is 6 to 10 years depending on the specialty. Some physicians, however, are grandfathered out of MOC requirements depending on their specialty and year of initial certification.

Accreditation and Certification Organizations

All education components along the path to becoming a practicing physician involve accreditation or licensure. Allopathic and osteopathic medical schools have their own accrediting organizations—the Liaison Committee on Medical Education (LCME) and the American Osteopathic Association (AOA) Commission on Osteopathic College Accreditation, respectively. In 2007, 129 accredited medical schools enrolled 17,759 first-year students (AAMC 2008a); 25 accredited osteopathic schools enrolled 4,528 first-year students (AACOM 2009). Accreditation standards for these schools cover a wide range of requirements, including clerkship setting requirements, education curricula, and educational resources.

Residency programs may be accredited by the ACGME or the AOA, or they may be dually accredited. In the 2007–2008 academic year, there were a total of 8,589 ACGME-approved residency programs, with 106,012 residents and fellows—an increase of 7.9 percent from the 2002–2003 academic year. The number of first-year residents totaled 23,759, an increase of 8.7 percent from five years earlier. International medical graduates accounted for 28.6 percent of first-year enrollment (Brotherton and Etzel 2008). In the 2007–2008 academic year, there were 223 AOA-approved internships and 718 AOA-approved residency programs with 4,934 osteopathic residents (Freeman and Lischka 2009).

Completing an accredited residency program is important for a number of reasons. All states, for example, require completion of a minimum number of years of an accredited residency before being granted a license to practice independently. Medicare also requires residency programs to be accredited to receive medical education funds from Medicare.[7] Finally, physicians must complete an accredited residency program to be eligible for board certification in a specialty. The text box (pp. 14–15) describes the process ACGME uses for residency program accreditation.

Although medical school, graduate medical education, and specialty certification are governed by separate accrediting agencies, many of their appointees come from some of the same pool of medical organizations (Table 1-2). For example, the American Medical Association and the Association of American Medical Colleges appoint members to the bodies that accredit medical schools (LCME) and residency programs (ACGME). Specialty groups are represented in the residency review committees (RRCs), which also govern specialty certification decisions for physicians. Some of the specialty boards have worked closely with the ACGME and RRCs in developing some of the changes that have taken place in the accreditation process. The groups represented in these accrediting agencies are also closely involved in providing undergraduate, graduate, and continuing medical education, including teaching hospitals and physician educators.

The interrelatedness of these organizations creates both benefits and concerns. Overlaps of the governance of these organizations for multiple purposes can help ensure some consistency and logical flow across the different points of the medical education continuum. However, the interrelatedness of accrediting bodies and their potential incentives for maintaining the status quo raise some concerns about reforming medical education policies. Several experts and researchers have discussed the possible role of an independent board in making decisions about allocating funding for medical education (COGME 2007, IOM 2003, Pew Center for Health Professions 1998, Whitcomb 2007). Another option is to increase the share of public members participating in the governance of these accrediting and certifying organizations.

Medicare's Subsidies for Graduate Medical Education

Since its inception, Medicare has subsidized much of graduate medical education in the United States. When the Congress created Medicare in 1965, it recognized the societal benefits of medical education and specified that the Medicare program support its share of medical education costs, until the community determined other means.

> Educational activities enhance the quality of care in an institution, and it is intended, until the community undertakes to bear such education costs in some other way, that a part of the net cost of such activities (including stipends of trainees, as well as compensation of teachers and other costs) should be considered as an element in the cost of patient care, to be borne to an appropriate extent by the hospital insurance program (U.S. House 1965, U.S. Senate 1965).

Currently, Medicare's subsidy is provided through both direct and indirect payments to teaching hospitals. In total, Medicare's payments for graduate medical education account for about $9 billion annually—an average of almost $100,000 per resident.

Payments toward Direct and Indirect Costs

Direct graduate medical education (GME) payments are designed to fund the teaching aspects of residency programs—resident salaries and benefits, supervisory physician salaries, and administrative overhead expenses. Direct GME payments are based on a hospital-specific per resident payment amount for which Medicare pays its share.

Table1-2. Multiple accrediting organizations are involved in physician education and practice

	Type of certification/accreditation				
	Medical school	**graduate medical education**	**Specialty certification**	**State licensure**	**Continuing medical education**
Accrediting organization	LCME	ACGME	ABMS	State medical boards	ACCME
Purpose	Accreditation of medical schools.	Accreditation of GME programs and institutions sponsoring GME programs.	Assist member boards in developing standards for certification of physicians in a given specialty.	License physicians, investigate complaints, and discipline physicians who violate the law.	Sets standards and accredits organizations andinstitutions that offer CME.
Governance	*17 members:* • 6 AAMC • 6 AMA • 2 students • 2 public • 1 CACMS	*25 members:* • 4 AAMC • 4 AHA • 4 AMA • 4 ABMS • 4 CMSS • 3 residents • 2 public • 1 government observer	*27 members:* • 1 from each specialty board • 3 public	Volunteer physicians and members of the public, in most cases, appointed by the governor. Total of 57 state medical boards.	*17 members:* • 3 AAMC • 3 ABMS • 3 AHA • 3 AMA • 1 AHME • 3 CMSS • 1 FSMB

Table1-2. (Continued)

	Medical school	graduate medical education	Specialty certification	State licensure	Continuing medical education
Related organizations	**ECFMG** Certifies eligibility of graduates of non-LCME accredited medical schools. *Members from:* • AAMC • ABMS • AHME • AMA • FSMB • NMA	**RRCs** Develop specialty-specific guidelines for accreditation. 24 separate RRCs for each major specialty. *Members from:* • AMA • Specialty boards • Specialty societies	**Specialty boards** Develop guidelines for certification and recertification.24 separate boards for each major specialty. *Members:*Physicians distinguished in teaching, research, or patient care	**FSMB** Cosponsors USMLE exam. Verifies physician credentials and maintains data bank on disciplinary actions. *Members from:* 57 state medical boards	**State medical societies** Approve state-specific CME *Members:*Individual physicians in a state.

Note: LCME (Liaison Committee on Medical Education), ACGME (Accreditation Council for Graduate Medical Education), ABMS (American Board of Medical Specialties), ACCME (Accreditation Council for Continuing Medical Education), GME (graduate medical education), CME (continuing medical education), AAMC (Association of American Medical Colleges), AMA (American Medical Association), CACMS (Committee on the Accreditation of Canadian Medical Schools), AHA (American Hospital Association), CMSS (Council of Medical Specialty Societies), AHME (Association for Hospital Medical Education), FSMB (Federation of State Medical Boards of the U.S., Inc.), ECFMG (Educational Commission on Foreign Medical Graduates), NMA (National Medical Association), RRC (residency review committee), USMLE (United States Medical Licensing Examination).

Source: MedPAC analysis of information from each of the accrediting organization’s public websites.

These payments, which go to teaching hospitals, totaled $2.9 billion in 2007. See the text box (pp. 16–17) for more details on Medicare's direct GME payment.

Medicare also provides a small amount of education funding to hospitals to support direct costs of hospital- based education and training programs for nursing and various allied health professions.[8] In future work, the Commission may examine ways to provide more support for nursing education, as nurses are key professionals in delivering coordinated patient care.

The indirect medical education (IME) adjustment is a percentage increase (or "add-on") to the inpatient prospective payment system rate that varies with the intensity of hospitals' residency programs. The IME adjustment was developed to account for the higher costs of patient care associated with care in teaching hospitals, such as unmeasured patient severity, residents "learning by doing," and greater use of emerging technologies. Because Medicare's IME payments are tied to Medicare inpatients, teaching hospitals in communities with smaller shares of Medicare beneficiaries receive proportionately lower total IME payments per resident.

When an IME adjustment was developed for Medicare's inpatient prospective payment system in 1983, it was set at double the empirical relationship between teaching intensity and costs per case, based on analysis estimating that teaching hospitals would not perform well financially under the new prospective payment system (Lave 1985). With the doubled adjustment, however, teaching hospitals performed much better than other hospitals. Despite some reductions in the IME adjustment over time, the Commission's analysis has shown that the current IME adjustment of 5.5 percent is set at more than twice the estimated relationship between teaching intensity and costs per cases (MedPAC 2007). In 2007, IME payments totaled $6.0 billion. The text box (pp. 16–17) provides additional details on Medicare's IME adjustment.

Summary of the Accreditation Council for Graduate Medical Education Residency Program Accreditation Process

The Accreditation Council for Graduate Medical Education (ACGME) accredits individual residency programs and the institution sponsoring the programs. The work of reviewing the programs and making accreditation decisions is carried out by 27 residency review committees (RRCs), 1 for each major specialty and 1 for transitional year programs. An institutional review committee accredits the institutions that sponsor residency programs. RRC members are volunteer physicians appointed by the appropriate medical specialty organization, medical specialty board, and the American Medical Association Council on Medical Education.

ACGME field staff representatives conduct one-day site visits to programs once every two to five years, depending on the strength of the program. They visit about one-third of the programs in a given year. The field staff representatives produce reports on the programs they visit based on lengthy interviews with program directors, faculty, and residents as well as a review of supporting documents. The RRCs, which on average meet three times a year, review the site visitors' reports along with data provided by the programs. The RRC members then vote on the appropriate accreditation action to take for each program on the agenda for that meeting.

Program Requirements

To meet accreditation standards, programs must fulfill the requirements set up by the RRCs for the individual specialties. The ACGME has established a set of common program requirements or general competencies that all programs are required to integrate into their curriculum: patient care, medical knowledge, practice-based learning and improvement, interpersonal and communication skills, professionalism, and systems-based practice. (The text box on pp. 20–21 describes these subject areas.)

The movement to a competency-based system of accreditation is part of the Outcome Project, a longterm initiative that started in 1999, by which the ACGME is increasing emphasis on educational outcome assessment in the accreditation process. The shift in emphasis to outcome assessment is reflected in requirements for programs to:

- identify learning objectives related to the ACGME general competencies,
- use increasingly more dependable (i.e., objective) methods of assessing residents' attainment of these competency-based objectives, and
- use outcome data to facilitate continuous improvement of both resident and residency program performance (ACGME 2008).

The Outcome Project is now in its third phase, which began in 2006, with full integration of the competencies and their assessment with learning and clinical care. The fourth phase, which will begin in 2011, will be an expansion of the competencies and their assessments to develop models of excellence, by identifying benchmark programs and adopting generalizable information about emerging models of excellence (ACGME 2008). The ACGME is also moving toward an evaluation system for programs that would be annual rather than every five years (Nasca 2008).

Before the Outcome Project, graduate medical education accreditation was based on a "minimal threshold model," by which programs were judged according to how they complied with minimum standards established by the RRCs and the ACGME. In the Outcome Project's competency-based model, programs are asked to show how residents have achieved competency-based educational objectives and, in turn, how programs use information drawn from evaluation of those objectives to improve the educational experience of the residents (ACGME 2008).

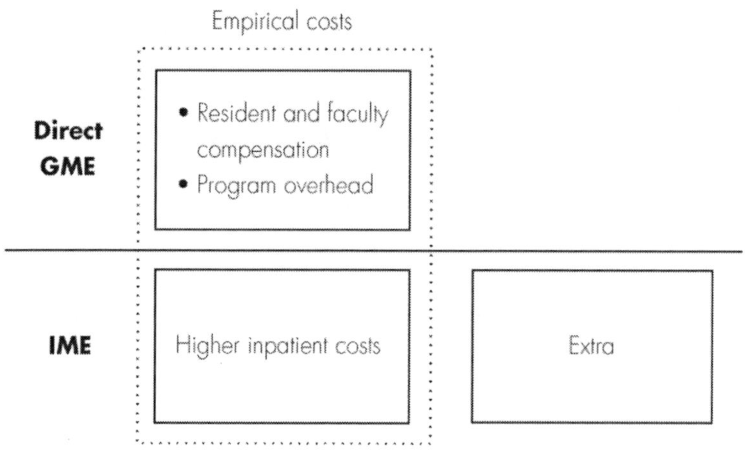

Note: GME (graduate medical education), IME (indirect medical education). "Extra" refers to the aggregate amount of IME payments that exceed empirically calculated IME costs.

Figure 1-3. Current Medicare subsidies for graduate medical education

The sum of Medicare's graduate medical education payments can be divided into three components, as illustrated in Figure 1-3. Two components reflect empirical costs discussed earlier: the cost of operating residency programs and the higher costs of patient care associated with educating and training residents. The third component is the extra IME payment that remains because the IME add-on is set at a percentage more than twice what can be empirically justified. In past reports, the Commission has recommended that part of the extra payment for IME be used to support a pay-for-performance program for all hospitals. The other two components—the direct GME and the empirically based portion of the IME payment— could be affected by policies that target funding to the type of settings and educational programs that best meet our health care needs.

Number of Residents that Medicare Supports

In 2006, Medicare provided direct GME support to hospitals for about 89,600 full-time equivalent (FTE) residents and fellows.[9] On average, hospitals received more than $70,000 in IME payments and $30,000 in direct GME payments for each FTE resident eligible for Medicare funding. Regulations for counting eligible FTEs for direct GME and IME payments are complex and vary, so the numbers Medicare supports through direct GME and IME payments differ. For the IME payment adjustment, Medicare supported 79,800 FTE residents in inpatient prospective payment system hospitals. For each teaching hospital, Medicare limits the number of residency positions it supports through a hospital-specific cap on medical education subsidies. However, hospitals may hire additional residents; in 2006, hospitals had more than 8,000 FTE residents for whom they did not have Medicare funding because the hospitals had exceeded their Medicare cap.[10] Preliminary research using cost report data suggests that hospitals that exceed Medicare's cap have a smaller proportion of residents in primary care specialties than hospitals that do not exceed the cap.

Non-Medicare Funding Sources for Graduate Medical Education

The aggregate spending from all payers for graduate medical education is not well known (Wynn et al. 2006). Although Medicare is the largest single contributor to graduate medical education, other funding sources exist, mostly through federal and state programs. For example, state Medicaid programs contribute more than $3 billion annually to graduate medical education financing. In addition, the Department of Veterans Affairs (VA) supports more than 9,000 resident FTEs and allows more than 30,000 residents and fellows to rotate through its hospitals each year. The Department of Defense supports the education and training of about 3,000 residents. The Children's Hospital Medical Education Program administered by the Health Resources and

Services Administration (HRSA) provides $300 million to support direct and indirect GME costs. Some Title VII grants administered by HRSA are also used to support residency programs in primary care and geriatrics, but funding for these programs is relatively low and has been reduced in recent years.

Teaching hospitals may also receive resources from their medical school affiliations, research grants, endowments, and foundation grants. Some private insurers contribute to supporting graduate medical education indirectly through higher patient care payments provided to teaching- affiliated health care providers. A small number of states require private insurers to contribute explicitly to graduate medical education. However, in most states private insurers generally do not make specific payments to providers for direct or indirect medical education costs.

Medicare Payments for Direct Graduate Medical Education (GME) and Indirect Medical Education (IME)

Direct GME Payments

Direct GME payments are based on hospital-specific per resident costs in a base period, updated each year for inflation by the consumer price index for all urban consumers (CPI-U). A hospital's payment is the product of three factors:

- the hospital's updated per resident payment amount;
- a weighted count of full-time equivalent residents supported by the facility; and
- the hospital's Medicare patient share, based on the ratio of Medicare patient days to total patient days in the acute inpatient setting.

Medicare direct GME payments totaled about $2.9 billion in 2007. Medicare makes direct GME payments to short-stay acute care hospitals as well as other types of hospitals supported by the Medicare program (cancer, children's, long-term care, psychiatric, and rehabilitation hospitals).

Hospitals' per resident payment amounts are based on their total per resident costs in 1984 updated for inflation. A floor rate was set at 85 percent of a locality-adjusted national average under the Medicare,

Medicaid, and SCHIP Benefits Improvement and Protection Act of 2000, which also eliminated annual CPI-U increases in the rates from 2001 through 2013 if a hospital's per resident amount is 140 percent or more of the locality-adjusted national average. The per resident payment amounts also depend on the residents' specialties. Payments are about 6 percent higher for residents in primary care specialties (family practice, general internal medicine, general pediatrics, and obstetrics and gynecology) and some selected specialties (geriatrics and public health and preventive medicine) than for other specialties. There is no differential in payments by specialty for hospitals that established residency programs after 1995 or for hospitals that are at the floor rate.

The weighted count of residents used in the payment formula is based on a three-year rolling average. The resident counts for most hospitals are also capped at their 1996 levels because of concern that the payment formulas were providing a strong incentive for hospitals to increase the number of residents in their programs.[11] Residents in their initial residency period—the minimum period required for board certification in the first specialty program entered after medical school, up to a maximum of five years—are given a weight of 1.0. Residents who pursue a second specialty or a subspecialty or who spend longer in their initial residency period are given a weight of 0.5.

A hospital's Medicare patient share is the proportion of its Medicare acute care inpatient days to its total acute care inpatient days. The formula for direct GME payments for Medicare Advantage patients is the same, but the Medicare patient share is based on Medicare Advantage patient days to total days.

IME Payments

The IME adjustment is a percentage add-on to a hospital's inpatient prospective payment system payments that varies with the intensity of the hospital's residency programs. The IME adjustment is currently set so that operating payments increase approximately 5.5 percent for each 10 percent increment in resident intensity, measured by the ratio of residents to hospital beds.[13] Because IME payments are an adjustment to base payment rates, a hospital's IME payments are tied to its volume and mix of Medicare cases as well as its number of residents. As is the case with direct GME payments, the number of residents included in the resident-to-bed ratio is also capped. Medicare IME payments totaled $6.0 billion in 2007.

While the IME adjustment is intended in part to pay for the indirect costs of running a teaching program, the current IME adjustment of 5.5 percent substantially exceeds the estimated relationship between teaching intensity and costs per case. The Commission's analysis has shown that Medicare inpatient costs per case (operating and capital costs combined) increase about 2.2 percent for every 10 percent increase in the ratio of residents to hospital beds (MedPAC 2007). The current IME adjustment is thus set at more than twice what can be empirically justified, directing more than $3 billion in extra payments to teaching hospitals above the effect that educating and supervising residents and fellows has on the cost of caring for Medicare patients. These funds are currently provided to teaching hospitals without any restriction on how they are used; teaching hospitals report that they use this extra payment amount for mission-driven activities, such as trauma-center care. To encourage quality improvement, the Commission believes some of these funds should be made available to all hospitals that provide high-quality care. The Commission therefore recommended in its 2007, 2008, and 2009 March reports that the IME adjustment be reduced from 5.5 percent to 4.5 percent per 10 percent increment in the resident-to-bed ratio and that the funds obtained from reducing the IME adjustment be used to help finance quality-incentive payments.

Medicare Payments to Teaching Physicians for Services when Supervising Residents

When supervising residents, teaching physicians are permitted to bill Medicare for Part B services that their residents perform. Residents may not bill for these services.[12] For payment, Medicare requires that the supervising physician be physically present during the critical or key portion of the service being provided or actually perform this portion of the service. In addition, the supervising physician must supply more than his or her signature in the clinical documentation for the service. Specifically, the supervising physician must document who provided what portions of the service and that the supervisor was present during the critical or key portion of the service and participated in management of the patient. These regulations apply to services provided under Medicare's physician fee schedule in hospital and nonhospital settings. In certain circumstances, Medicare relaxes the supervision requirements for primary care services but increases the requirements for surgical, high- risk, or other complex procedures.

In the middle to late 1990s the Department of Health and Human Services' Office of Inspector General undertook a series of audits of physician services at teaching hospitals. These were called the Payment for Academic Teaching Hospitals (PATH) audits. Since they took place, CMS and teaching hospitals have increased their focus on ensuring compliance with the supervision rules.

Economic Costs and Benefits of Participating in Teaching Activities

To varying degrees, participation in graduate medical education provides both costs and benefits to hospitals and physicians. With respect to direct costs, teaching hospitals incur the expenses associated with operating a residency program, including salary and benefit costs of residents, faculty supervisory costs, and program overhead expenses. Other types of costs include facility infrastructure expenses, such as maintaining an extensive medical library for residents to conduct clinical research, providing office space for supervisory faculty, providing on-call rooms for residents, and adopting expensive technologies. Teaching hospitals also experience added indirect costs such as higher costs of patient care from residents learning by doing, from ordering more services (e.g., diagnostic tests and imaging), and from taking longer to perform procedures.

Alternatively, teaching hospitals benefit in many ways from having residents, and overall the number of residents in accredited programs has increased 30 percent during the last two decades (Salsberg et al. 2008). Benefits to teaching hospitals include, for example, Medicare and Medicaid payments to hospitals toward the direct and indirect costs of residency programs described earlier. Moreover, Medicare's indirect payments are currently set so hospitals receive payments that are more than double the indirect costs. Hospitals also benefit by having residents available for on-call coverage and to assist in providing patient care. In many cases, resident wages are lower than those of other health professionals who could perform these duties, thus affording hospitals some gains in staffing costs (Rich et al. 2002). Teaching hospitals and affiliated physicians also benefit from the prestige associated with being involved in physician education and training. The last two factors— greater physician staffing and prestige—can lead to higher patient volumes, as patients and community physicians favor these facilities. With prestige may also come the ability to garner higher prices in negotiations from private payers to help cover these institutions' higher costs for patient care.

Similarly, physicians experience costs and benefits from their participation in medical education. Depending on the resident's skill level, a supervising physician's productivity may fall because of the extra time needed for activities such as teaching and reviewing clinical documentation with residents. Recent actions regarding medical education—such as rules restricting residents' duty hours to 80 per week and the PATH audits—may have decreased residents' and supervisory physician's output, but research on this topic is limited. One study on surgery showed that surgical operations take longer with resident involvement (Babineau et al. 2004). Another study of residents in an internal medicine practice showed small productivity losses from participating in residency instruction, more so for first-year residents (Johnson et al. 2008).[14] Other supervisory costs include the time involved in negotiating agreements and maintaining paperwork on individual residents. Some practices also incur costs from expanding office space to accommodate residents in their office.

Experienced physicians can also benefit from participation in residency supervision and education. Many are paid by the teaching hospital for their role in educational, supervisory, and administrative activities. Even when physicians volunteer their time, they may receive a faculty appointment, which adds prestige to their practice and may also allow access to other benefits from the educational sponsor, such as medical library privileges. Faculty appointments may help increase practice volume and total patient revenues. In addition, being involved in medical education allows physicians to keep up with the latest medical research and provides an opportunity to recruit future practice partners. Residents may also help with on-call coverage in physician practices as well as patient preparation and triage—thereby increasing the practice's productivity.

Given the complexities of calculating the costs and benefits of participating in GME, it is difficult to discern whether it is, on net, profitable for providers. Hospitals' and physicians' decision to participate in GME activities may also be driven by their mission focus, such as education and research.

Medical Education should Support Needed Delivery System Reform

Our health care delivery system is not a true system: care coordination across providers is not routine, fragmented specialist care is often favored over primary care, quality of care is too often poor, and costs are high and increasing at an unsustainable rate. In congressional testimony and in our reports to the Congress, the Commission calls for payment system reforms and other tools to moderate spending while increasing value. To this end, the Commission has recommended the following changes aimed at encouraging physicians to increase care coordination and assume greater accountability for quality and resource use:

- medical home pilot programs for beneficiaries with multiple chronic conditions,
- efforts to measure physicians' use of health care resources and provide feedback results,
- financial disincentives for certain hospital readmissions,
- pilot program for bundled payments for all services provided in a hospitalization episode,
- linking providers' payment to quality, and
- encouraging the use of comparative-effectiveness information and public reporting.

Such reforms in payment policies need to be accompanied by reforms in medical education. This pairing is important to ensure that students and residents learn the skills they need to provide care and leadership in new delivery models under restructured payment and incentives.

These skills include quality measurement and practice improvement, care coordination, multidisciplinary teamwork, cost awareness, and interpersonal skills. Research on internal medicine residency programs (discussed later in this chapter) found several gaps in formal instruction on many of these skills.

Residency experiences are designed to prepare physicians for clinical practices. Thus, exposure to skills such as care coordination during residencies is critical to improving the quality and efficiency of our nation's health care. Recognizing shortcomings, the specialties of internal medicine, family medicine, surgery, and pediatrics have embarked on major redesigns of their residency programs to improve the way residents prepare for practice in their specialty (Whitcomb 2008). Further, recent ACGME requirements in residency program curricula (described in text box, pp. 20–21) also seek to address some of these concerns.

Yet, Medicare—with an enormous financial stake in health care and graduate medical education—has never specifically linked any of its direct GME or IME subsidies to promoting or fostering important goals in medical education. Medicare should consider ways to ensure that residents and other health care professionals obtain the skills they need to provide efficient, coordinated, high- quality care.

Study Suggests that Curricula in Many Internal Medicine Residency Programs Fall Short in Topics Associated with Delivery System Reform

A Commission-sponsored study, conducted by RAND researchers, found that, although most internal medicine residency programs provide at least some instruction and experience in topics associated with quality and efficiency improvements, their curricula fall short of recommendations from the Institute of Medicine (IOM) and other experts (Cordasco et al. 2009).[15] This study consisted of semistructured interviews with 26 directors from a representative sample of internal medicine residency programs. It examined several specific formal and experiential curricular activities within the following broad topics:

- practice-based learning, focusing on measuring care quality and improving medical practice;
- system-based practice, focusing on care coordination, multi-isciplinary teamwork, cost awareness, and patient safety;
- interpersonal communication, focusing on communication with other providers, patients, and family and on patient education;
- health information technology, including electronic medical records and computer order entry; and
- care settings, focusing on experiences in nonhospital settings.

Of particular concern from the interview findings is the lack of formal instruction and experience in: multidisciplinary teamwork, cost awareness in clinical decision making, comprehensive health information technology, and patient care in ambulatory settings. Formal instruction involves structured and organized educational experiences. Topics that residency program directors reported to be covered with more consistency through formal instruction are evidence-based medicine and communicating with patients about end-of-life care. In all areas, particularly interpersonal communication, directors reported that more experiential learning—with faculty modeling, mentoring, and informal feedback—is the predominant form of instruction. As may be expected, researchers found large variation in the extent of and approach to teaching these topics, and program directors reported multiple factors that facilitated or impeded their ability to instruct residents in them.

The project consisted of 26 hour-long telephone interviews with program directors from a representative, random sample of internal medicine programs.[16] A board-certified internal medicine physician, familiar with residency education, conducted all interviews. Given available resources, we were unable to expand the scope of this project to include other types of residency programs, such as family medicine and surgical programs. It is likely that findings would differ among specialties.

Practice-Based Learning: Measuring Care Quality and Improving Medical Practice

The IOM states that physicians must be able to assess the quality of care they provide and implement changes in their practice for improvement. This process is often referred to as practice-based learning and calls for physicians to obtain skills in two aspects: the methodology of quality measurement and the use of tools for implementing practice or system changes where quality is deficient (Ogrine et al. 2003). Systematic data collection and the use of chronic disease registries provide educational and experiential opportunities for obtaining experience in quality measurement. The American Board of Internal Medicine offers a web-based learning module on collecting patient data and implementing practice changes. Experience with tools such as evidence-based medicine and clinical decision aids are geared toward improving practice and systems.

THE ACCREDITATION COUNCIL FOR GRADUATE MEDICAL EDUCATION (ACGME) COMMON PROGRAM REQUIREMENTS: GENERAL COMPETENCIES

Approved by the ACGME Board February 13, 2007

ACGME Competencies

The program must integrate the following ACGME competencies into the curriculum:

Patient Care

Residents must be able to provide patient care that is compassionate, appropriate, and effective for the treatment of health problems and the promotion of health.

Medical Knowledge

Residents must demonstrate knowledge of established and evolving biomedical, clinical, epidemiological, and social–behavioral sciences as well as the application of this knowledge to patient care.

Practice-based Learning and Improvement

Residents must demonstrate the ability to investigate and evaluate their care of patients, to appraise and assimilate scientific evidence, and to continuously improve patient care based on constant self-evaluation and lifelong learning. Residents are expected to develop skills and habits to be able to meet the following goals:

- identify strengths, deficiencies, and limits in one's knowledge and expertise.
- set learning and improvement goals.
- identify and perform appropriate learning activities.
- systematically analyze practice using quality improvement methods, and implement changes with the goal of practice improvement.
- incorporate formative evaluation feedback into daily practice.
- locate, appraise, and assimilate evidence from scientific studies related to their patients' health problems.
- use information technology to optimize learning.
- participate in the education of patients, families, students, residents, and other health professionals.

Interpersonal and Communication Skills

Residents must demonstrate interpersonal and communication skills that result in the effective exchange of information and collaboration with patients, their families, and health professionals. Residents are expected to:

- communicate effectively with patients, families, and the public, as appropriate, across a broad range of socioeconomic and cultural backgrounds.
- communicate effectively with physicians, other health professionals, and health-related agencies.
- work effectively as a member or leader of a health care team or other professional group.
- act in a consultative role to other physicians and health professionals.
- maintain comprehensive, timely, and legible medical records, if applicable.

Professionalism

Residents must demonstrate a commitment to carrying out professional responsibilities and an adherence to ethical principles. Residents are expected to demonstrate:

- compassion, integrity, and respect for others;
- responsiveness to patient needs that supersedes self- interest;
- respect for patient privacy and autonomy;
- accountability to patients, society, and the profession; and
- sensitivity and responsiveness to a diverse patient population, including but not limited to diversity in gender, age, culture, race, religion, disabilities, and sexual orientation.

Systems-based Practice

Residents must demonstrate an awareness of and responsiveness to the larger context and system of health care as well as the ability to call effectively on other resources in the system to provide optimal health care. Residents are expected to:

- work effectively in various health care delivery settings and systems relevant to their clinical specialty.
- coordinate patient care within the health care system relevant to their clinical specialty.
- incorporate considerations of cost awareness and risk–benefit analysis in patient or population-based care as appropriate.
- advocate for quality patient care and optimal patient care systems.
- work in interprofessional teams to enhance patient safety and improve patient care quality.
- participate in identifying system errors and implementing potential systems solutions.

The RAND researchers found that, while many residency programs provide some exposure to quality assurance and system change, only a small share require residents to complete their own systematic data collection, analysis, and resulting system change (Table 1-3, p. 22). Fewer than half the programs (11 of 26 programs) have lectures or computer-based training on quality assurance, but more (18 programs) require that residents work on quality assessment at the hospital. Fewer than a third (seven programs) have established curricula in which residents collect and analyze data on their own patients. The same share of programs introduces residents to chronic disease registries and provides lectures or computer-based training on implementing system change. Fewer still (four programs) have residents work directly on projects to implement system changes.

Among the programs in the study that seem to devote more resident time to quality measurement and practice improvement, one includes requiring these activities throughout an ambulatory rotation that spans several months. In some programs, a hospital's quality management department co-leads efforts in these curricula.

Overall, program directors reported that their residents' instruction in evidence-based medicine is stronger. The most frequent instruction methods in this topic are formal sessions on how to search and conduct literature reviews and journal article discussions.

Table 1-3. Residency instruction in measuring quality and improving medical practice

Topic/activity	Number of programs (of 26) that include topic in curricula
QA and improvement	
Have lectures/computer-based training in QA	11
Hospital administration collects, analyzes, and presents data to residents on quality measures	9
Each resident works on quality assessment	1 8
Residents collect or are provided data on own patients	7
Use chronic disease registries	7
Have lectures/computer-based training in system change implementation	7
Each resident does project implementing system change	4
EBM	
Formal session—searching literature	18
Journal club/EBM conference	26
Lectures on critiquing literature	13
EBM assignments	8
Clinical decision aids	
Use order sets or critical pathways	18
Formal lectures on clinical prediction tools	6
IT supports clinical prediction tools	9

Note: QA (quality assurance), EBM (evidence-based medicine), IT (information technology). Table presents presence but not intensity level of the activity.
Source: Cordasco et al. 2009.

Half the programs provide residents with faculty mentoring or assistance from an epidemiologist or statistician for literature analysis. Most program directors reported that evidence-based medicine is also taught informally through daily interactions with faculty in the course of patient care. While most programs reported teaching their residents to use clinical prediction rules (e.g., pneumonia severity index), only a little more than one-third (nine programs) have information technology to support these tools in clinical practice. In some cases, however, residents have the technology on their personal hand-held computers.

System-Based Practice: Care Coordination, Cost Awareness, and Patient Safety

Individual physicians work within a complex arrangement of health care delivery in the United States. This complexity has led to fragmentation in care along the continuum of health care services (within a hospitalization, at hospital discharge, and in outpatient care). Moreover, discontinuity has likely contributed to the increase in hospitalizations that researchers have found are related to exacerbations or complications of chronic conditions (Wolff et al. 2002). To counter this trend and the unsustainable growth in health care spending, experts have introduced system-based practice, which calls for a better understanding of the components and costs of health care delivery to improve coordination, spending, and safety (Berwick 1996). Under this concept, physicians— regardless of their practice setting—must be able to coordinate plans of care, work with multidisciplinary professionals, and utilize systems ensuring patient safety (Shortell et al. 2000).

RAND researchers found that formal instruction on many aspects of system-based practice is limited or nonexistent, particularly in the outpatient setting (Table 1-4). For the inpatient setting, program directors stated that coordinating provider handoffs of patients has recently become an area of increased attention in residency programs. Many programs (14 programs) have specific instruction in handoffs and some (6 programs) have supervision in "sign- out" procedures to communicate inpatient status during the residents' shift changes. For coordinating care across hospital discharge, the experience is less formalized, with fewer than half (11 programs) having formal instruction on this activity. Among those that do, case managers often lead the instruction. One program reported that residents rotate through a special "discharge team" that takes the lead on care coordination and patient education on the day of discharge. Compared with the inpatient setting, formal care coordination instruction for the outpatient setting is even less common. Fewer than one-third (eight programs) reported that their residents receive specific instruction or attend conferences on care coordination in the outpatient setting.

Table 1-4. Residency instruction in care coordination, cost awareness, and safety

Topic/activity	Number of programs (of 26) that include topic in curricula
Coordination of care	
Formal instruction in inpatient provider hand-offs	14
Faculty/chief resident supervise sign-outs	6
IT support (computer-based tool) for sign-outs	10
Formal instruction in hospital discharge coordination	11
IT supports hospital discharge	14
Formal instruction in outpatient coordination	8
IT supports outpatient coordination	11
Multidisciplinary teams	
Formal inpatient teams	19
Formal teams on general medical inpatient service	4
Formal outpatient teams	8
Awareness of absolute and relative costs	
Lectures on costs/cost-effectiveness	6
Lectures on patient share of costs	6
Patient safety issues/methods	
Formal instruction in patient safety issues	26
Formal instruction on safety design principles	6
Patient safety project	4

Note: IT (information technology). Table identifies presence but not intensity level of the activity. Programs without formal multidisciplinary training may have semiformal or informal experiences.

Source: Cordasco et al. 2009.

Similarly, formal experience working in multidisciplinary teams (often composed of physicians, nurses, social workers, nutritionists, and pharmacists) is more common in the inpatient setting than in the outpatient setting. Of the 19 programs with formal inpatient multidisciplinary team experience, most are on subspecialty rotations; only 4 programs include formal multidisciplinary teamwork during the general medicine service rotation. Fewer than one-third (eight programs) reported formal multidisciplinary experience in the outpatient setting, but directors from these programs often noted that residents may engage in semiformal or informal multidisciplinary teamwork or have multidisciplinary staff available for consultation.

Only about one-quarter (six programs) have formal methods for teaching about absolute and relative costs of diagnostic tests, treatments, and medications. Most program directors indicated that they rely on informal instruction for this topic. Among those that have formal instruction, directors mentioned topics such as hospital service costs, billing, and coding. Programs are similarly unlikely to instruct residents about patients' share of medical charges. Among those that do, the focus is typically during ambulatory experiences, such as in a clinic that uses sliding-scale policies. Directors did not mention having formal instruction about overall spending on health care in their residency programs, but the study did not ask about it specifically.[17]

All programs include some formal instruction in patient safety issues (e.g., preventing falls, proper patient identification). However, only about one-quarter (six programs) teach basic safety design principles, as recommended by the IOM. These principles include methods such as standardization of practices and analysis of the root causes of safety problems. Some (four programs) require residents to be involved in safety-related projects that examine causes of adverse or "near miss" events within the hospital.

Interpersonal Communication

The quality of communication between patients and their physicians is important, as aspects of care such as adherence to treatment regimens and satisfaction with care plans can influence patients' health outcomes (Lorig et al. 2001, Stewart et al. 2000). Thus, to maximize health care effectiveness, it is essential for physicians to communicate collaboratively with patients and their families as well as with other health professionals to determine appropriate diagnostic and treatment regimens. Instruction in this area should teach new physicians how to communicate with patients and families in ways that are adaptable to patient age, culture, health literacy, and health status. Communication skills are particularly important when treating patients with chronic illnesses because self-management of chronic diseases relies on patients' and caregivers' clear understanding of symptoms and treatment. Previous Commission work has highlighted the importance of physician communication with patients about end-of-life treatment choices and decisions (MedPAC 2008).

The RAND researchers in this study found that, although only a little more than half the programs (15 programs) cover communication skills between health care providers, more, but not all (22 programs), include formal instruction on how to communicate clearly with patients about diagnoses and treatment plans (Table 1-5, p. 24). Looking specifically at forms of patient–physician communication, we see that communication activities that include more patient engagement are less frequently included in formal residency instruction. For example, half the programs (13 programs) instruct residents on how to conduct shared decision making, only 10 formally instruct residents on how to counsel patients on regimen adherence and behavior change, and fewer than one-third (8 programs) ensure resident experience with the techniques of patient education, such as those used for the management of chronic disease (e.g., diabetes education classes).

Table 1-5. Residency instruction in interpersonal communication

Topic/activity	Number of programs (of 26) that include topic in curricula
Communication skills with health care providers	15
Communicating clearly with patients about diagnosis and treatment plan	22
Engaging patients in shared	
decision making	13
Patient education techniques	8
Counseling in adherence/behavior change	10
Cultural competency	24
Using interpreters	7
Health literacy	13
End-of-life communications	22
Holding family meetings on end-of-life issues	7

Note: Table identifies presence of formal training sessions about the topic but not intensity level of the communication activity. Programs without formal sessions may rely on informal instruction during patient care experiences.

Source: Cordasco et al. 2009.

With respect to instruction on communication with special populations or in special situations, most residency programs (24 programs) indicated that they have formal sessions on cultural competency, but only a little more than a quarter (7 programs) specifically teach skills for working with an interpreter.

Half (13 programs) provide instruction on adapting communication based on patients' health literacy. In most programs (22 programs), directors reported that residents receive formal instruction on how to communicate end-of-life issues, such as advance directives, with patients and caregivers. Only seven programs formally instruct residents on how to hold family meetings to discuss end-of-life issues.

Use of Health Information Technology

The use of information technology (IT) is a critical component of improving the quality, safety, and efficiency of health care delivery (MedPAC 2005). To make such improvements, physicians must become adept with the tools of infomatics, such as electronic medical records, computer order entry, electronic sources of medical care information and guidelines, and IT-supported clinical decision-making aids (Gorman et al. 2000, IOM 2003).

In recent legislation, the Congress included substantial financial incentives (totaling up to almost $37 billion from Medicare and Medicaid over the next 10 years) for hospitals and physicians to adopt health IT. To qualify for these incentive payments, providers must prove that their health IT is certified and that it is put to "meaningful use." Through the federal rule-making process, the Secretary of Health and Human Services will define the certification process and the term "meaningful use." To maximize federal (Medicare and Medicaid) investment in these IT incentives, it will be essential to ensure that participating hospitals and physicians commit to using the technology for improving the quality, efficiency, and safety of care. The Commission has recommended that performance incentives be based on the results gained through IT use, rather than simply the possession of health IT. Other key features for the success of health IT will be interoperability and standardization. Interoperability will facilitate the transfer of data and other communications across providers and settings. Standardization among technologies will allow professionals to know how to use health IT when they switch between settings. Even if health IT is standardized and interoperable, health care providers will still need to redesign some elements of their practice to take full advantage of this important technology.

In our study, the RAND researchers found that, although all interviewed programs provide residents with some exposure to electronic medical records (EMRs), in most programs, the EMRs are not comprehensive and lack one or more important components, such as the ability to enter orders or patient progress notes (Table 1-6). Only 1 of the 26 programs uses a comprehensive EMR in both inpatient and outpatient settings (not shown). Because the VA hospitals and clinics are equipped with comprehensive EMRs, residents who rotate through VA facilities gain some experience with high-functioning EMRs. Five programs reported that none of their residents' outpatient experiences includes the use of EMRs. The remaining programs include either comprehensive or partial EMR experience in the outpatient setting. As shown previously in Table 1-3, residency experience in using health IT to support other clinical functions (e.g., decision support and outpatient coordination) is limited.

Residency experience in nonhospital settings

Hospital inpatient experience is an important component of residency education to gain exposure to acute, serious illnesses, but it is equally essential for residents to have adequate experience in nonhospital settings. As has been documented over decades, most health care is provided in settings other than acute care hospitals (Green et al. 2001, White et al. 1961). Therefore, residents should receive sufficient education and training in nonhospital settings. Also, to coordinate care for patients across settings, residents need exposure to and experience in a variety of health care settings (COGME 1999, IOM 2003).

Table 1-6. Residency exposure to information technology

Setting and IT capability	Number of programs (of 26) that include IT capability in curricula
Inpatient	
Comprehensive EMR	4
Partial EMR	22
Computer order entry	11
Outpatient	
Comprehensive EMR	7
Partial EMR	14
Computer order entry	8

Note: IT (information technology), EMR (electronic medical record). Table identifies the presence but not the intensity level of the instruction in IT- related activities. Programs without formal sessions may rely on informal instruction during patient care experiences.

Source: Cordasco et al. 2009.

The RAND researchers found that the share of residents' time working in community-based medicine or in ambulatory settings with patients in managed care is extremely limited, even though most programs (21 programs) include at least some community clinic or private practice experiences in their residency. For most of these programs, directors reported that nonhospital experiences account for only a small amount of physicians' total residencies. About half the programs require residents to perform home visits and many require a rotation in which the residents provide care in a nursing home or rehabilitation unit (Table 1-7). Many directors reported that their residents have some experience with ambulatory patient populations in managed care, but in several of them, managed care patients were only a small share of the residents' caseloads. No directors reported that their residents have experience in a medical practice designated as a "medical home" by insurers or accrediting organizations; however, several directors indicated that their clinics are either working toward achieving this designation or have many of the features of one.

Teaching hospitals face considerable financial incentives and regulatory barriers that discourage them from rotating residents to nonhospital settings. We discuss these issues, as well as the impacts of residents' limited nonhospital experience, in a later section of this chapter.

Table 1-7. Residency experience in selected nonhospital settings

Setting	Number of programs (of 26) that include at least some experience in nonhospital setting
Community clinic or private practice	21
Home visits	14
Nursing homes or rehabilitation centers	21
Ambulatory care, managed care patients	20
Palliative care/hospice*	18

Note: Table presents ever/never experience in the setting but does not present information on the total time in the setting.

*Training in palliative care and hospice can occur in the hospital or nonhospital setting.

Source: Cordasco et al. 2009.

Factors Affecting Programs' Instruction in Selected Topics

During their interviews, residency program directors reported to the RAND researchers that multiple factors affect their ability to instruct in selected topics on practice- based learning, system-based practice, and interpersonal communication. These factors include IT infrastructure, faculty expertise and time, institutional support, the program's setting, residents' baseline characteristics, and relative lack of research-based evidence on the best methods for instructing residents on these skills.

The presence or absence of IT was the factor cited most often that either facilitated or impeded instruction in topics essential for delivery system reform. Directors stated that a comprehensive EMR system at residency sites was not only key for helping residents gain competence in using EMRs but was also helpful in teaching other skills. For example, EMRs provide data sources for quality improvement projects, tools for reinforcing the use of clinical decision support, methods to coordinate patient care between inpatient and outpatient settings, links to patient education materials, and, in some cases, comparative-effectiveness and cost information. We discussed opportunities and challenges related to health IT investments in a previous section of this chapter.

In the interviews, residency program directors stated that the levels of faculty expertise and institutional support (i.e., support from the sponsoring hospital) were key determinants of the quality and quantity of teaching in topics associated with delivery system reform. Directors often attributed the success of a given curriculum to a "faculty champion" who spearheaded its development and implementation. Alternatively, where curricula were lacking, directors cited weaker faculty members, among other contributing factors. They also noted that the attending physicians' clinical productivity requirements for the hospital can sometimes supersede the educational needs of the residency program. Competing with the hospital for the residents' time was frequently cited as a major barrier to teaching on topics relevant to delivery system reform, such as care coordination across settings. In contrast, programs with stronger institutional support for the residency programs—such as the availability of comprehensive health IT—appeared to have more ability to instruct on the topics we examined. Overall, directors viewed program accreditation requirements as being crucial for obtaining institutional support for their curriculum needs.

In discussion about facilitators and barriers, directors again raised the issue of care settings, indicating that opportunities and barriers may rest in the environment of the sponsoring hospital and community. For example, some programs serve a diverse patient population, but others do not. Some programs rely on rotations in community-based clinics that provide more experience with ambulatory care for lower income individuals, but placement in this type of setting was relatively rare.

Program directors also cited the level of residents' incoming knowledge from medical school as a factor in program strength. Directors generally indicated that physicians entered their residency with little experience in quality improvement methods but relatively stronger experience in evidence-based medicine skills. The variation in residents' skill levels in interpersonal communication was also cited as a major factor, particularly for international medical graduates. Directors also noted that residents' general lack of interest in these topics is a barrier, particularly because they are not a focus on board certification exams.

Finally, program directors reported a dearth of proven educational methods or tools available for teaching residents competencies in topics such as care coordination. Directors noted that it is difficult to determine the appropriate mix of formal and informal instruction methods because tools for evaluating their effectiveness are limited.

Study Limitations

This study presents a snapshot of the current activities and methods that internal medicine residency programs are using to instruct in topics important for reforming the U.S. health care delivery system. It does not provide a comprehensive analysis of each topic's educational methods because each topic could be the subject of its own study. Note that the absence or presence of teaching in a specific area is only a crude measure and does not represent curriculum quality, intensity, or effectiveness. Although our sample included only 26 of 381 (7 percent) internal medicine programs, the sampling frame was designed to produce a representative sample of internal medicine programs. In other specialties, it is likely that results would differ.

FINANCIAL INCENTIVES AND REGULATORY BARRIERS DISCOURAGE NONHOSPITAL RESIDENCY ROTATIONS

In keeping with historical patterns of graduate medical education, residency programs are largely based in inpatient, acute care teaching hospitals. Although this setting provides residents with important and crucial experience diagnosing and treating a variety of seriously ill patients, it is equally important for most residents to have adequate experience in nonhospital settings for a number of reasons.

First, as changes in health care have evolved, most of the medical conditions that practicing physicians confront are, and should be, managed in nonhospital settings, such as offices, nursing facilities, and patient homes. Thus, residents' education and training should include settings that will give them sufficient experience diagnosing and treating common medical problems and chronic conditions. Some research has found, for example, that internal medicine residents reported that they did not perform many common ambulatory procedures frequently enough (if at all) during their residencies and were, thus, not confident in performing them (Wickstrom et al. 2000). In other studies, family medicine residents were more likely to report feeling prepared for treating outpatients, whereas internal medicine residents were more likely to report feeling prepared to treat inpatients (Wiest et al. 2002). It is important for residents to be prepared to practice independently in nonhospital and outpatient settings because the complexity of patients and their care in these settings has grown.

Second, to understand how to coordinate care for patients across settings, residents need exposure to and experience in a variety of health care settings (COGME 2007, IOM 2004b). Third, improving residents' comfort level with care in these settings not only positively influences residents' skills in community-based care but could also increase their desire to practice community-based care—an essential component of a delivery system designed to prevent patients from being unnecessarily hospitalized. Taken together, these three reasons strongly suggest that enhancing residents' skills in nonhospital settings is important for patient health, patient comfort, and health care spending.

Currently, the relatively large share of residency time spent in hospital settings can be attributed to historical patterns of medical education, financial incentives, and regulatory issues. These factors encourage teaching hospitals to keep residents in the hospital and discourage hospitals from developing nonhospital rotations for their residents. We focus on the regulatory issues and the financial incentives in this section of the chapter.

Residents Provide Clinical Labor in Hospitals

For hospitals, residents provide valuable clinical services, particularly on-call duties that may include writing timely prescription orders and conducting patient admissions. Hiring or contracting other physicians, physician assistants, or nurse practitioners to provide these activities and services is more expensive for the hospital because hospitals must pay them higher wages (Rich et al. 2002). Moreover, Medicare does not subsidize the salaries and fringe benefits paid to these other health professionals, as it does for residents.

This labor cost incentive has been a longstanding constraint on hospitals' willingness to reduce residents' time in the inpatient setting, cited by many experts including the Commonwealth Fund Task Force on Academic Health Centers, the IOM Committee on the Roles of Academic Health Centers in the 21st Century, the Council on Graduate Medical Education, and the Blue Ridge Academic Health Group (Ludmerer and Johns 2005). Recent reductions in the limits on residents' total duty hours have intensified this incentive because hospitals have fewer hours per resident available.[18]

Table 1-8. Medicare supports didactic (nonpatient care) instruction in the hospital setting only

Site of residency instruction	Direct GME	IME
Teaching hospital	All approved educational activities: • Patient care activities • Didactic instruction (e.g., interdisciplinary grand rounds) • Research	Patient careactivities
Nonhospital setting*	Patient care activities	Patient care activities

Note: GME (graduate medical education), IME (indirect medical education). *Teaching hospitals must have a written agreement or other documents in place demonstrating that they are incurring the costs of residents' salary and benefits and all or substantially all of the nonhospital setting's supervisory activities.

Source: Adapted from Association of American Medical Colleges 2008d.

Medicare Supports Didactic (Nonpatient Care) Instruction in the Hospital Setting Only

Medicare's support for graduate medical education draws some distinctions regarding both the type of instructional experience and the setting (Table 1-8).

- IME payments are limited to activities that are specific to individual patient care. Thus, IME payments do not cover residents' time spent on research and didactic activities (e.g., a meeting or a lecture) that are unrelated to the care of residents' specific patients—regardless of the setting. Teaching hospitals can continue to receive IME payments for residents performing patient care activities in nonhospital settings.
- Direct GME can cover time related to residents' research and didactic (nonpatient care) learning experiences, but only when these experiences take place within the teaching hospital. Therefore, didactic activities that take place in nonhospital settings (e.g., meetings on overall practice management in physician offices) do not qualify for Medicare's direct GME payments.

Under these regulations, therefore, for each resident who rotates to a nonhospital setting, the teaching hospital effectively loses the resident's direct GME payment proportional to the time the resident spends in didactic (nonpatient care) activities. The teaching hospital also would not qualify for IME payments for these didactic activities, but that is true regardless of the setting.

To enforce this policy, teaching hospitals must track and characterize all their residents' hours as either patient care or otherwise at various sites and submit the information to Medicare in a log, which may be audited. The ACGME also requires this information to review completion of specialty requirements.

Additional Medicare statute and regulations require that teaching hospitals incur "all or substantially all" of the costs borne by nonhospital settings for teaching residents, including the cost of supervision. Thus, teaching hospitals must incur the costs of research and supervised didactic (nonpatient care) activities that occur in nonhospital settings. However, teaching hospitals do not receive direct GME payments for these non-patientcare activities when they occur outside the hospital. Consequently, under Medicare regulations, teaching hospitals must pay for the cost of research and didactic activities performed in nonhospital settings, when they are expressly excluded from Medicare's medical education subsidy.

Medicare Regulates Specific Provisions of Hospital–Nonhospital Residency Arrangements

If teaching hospitals do not show Medicare that they are incurring all or substantially all of the nonhospitals' costs related to resident teaching and supervision, they forgo direct GME and IME payments proportional to the time residents spend outside the hospital. Although some in nonhospital settings may welcome this compensation for their time, others would prefer to volunteer their time and are not willing to complete the paperwork that teaching hospitals need to comply with Medicare regulations. This paperwork includes a written agreement stating that the teaching hospital will incur the costs of the residents' salaries and fringe benefits in addition to the portion of the teaching physicians' salaries and fringe benefits attributable to resident instruction and supervision.[19] To fulfill these regulations, CMS would also accept written documentation proving such payments were made, in lieu of a formal written agreement.

Calculating the cost of this supervisory activity can be complex, and physician organizations, such as the American Association of Family Physicians, report that although CMS has taken some steps to reduce this paperwork burden, it is still cumbersome and many supervising physicians would prefer to volunteer their time.[20] Attending physicians enjoy mentoring new physicians, view it as a professional responsibility, and may often gain stature by being listed as "adjunct faculty" at the affiliated teaching institution. In addition, depending on the skills of the resident, nonhospital sites may gain in productivity with residents' patient care activities.

Without these written agreements or other documentation on the hospital's responsibility to incur all or substantially all of the costs of a resident's training in a nonhospital site, the teaching hospital effectively loses Medicare's graduate medical education payments for that resident's time in the nonhospital setting. With some exceptions, nonhospital settings are not permitted to receive direct GME and IME payments directly from Medicare.[21] Some have called for graduate medical education funding to go directly to more types of nonhospital entities responsible for providing the medical instruction and resident learning experiences (AAFP 2009, Mullan 2009, Rich et al. 2002).

As stated earlier, teaching hospitals that meet the regulations for claiming nonhospital resident time not only receive direct GME but also continue to receive IME payments for the time residents rotate in nonhospital settings, provided they are performing patient care (Table 1-7, p. 25). This allowance was instituted in the Balanced Budget Act of 1997 to ameliorate the financial disincentives for teaching hospitals to rotate residents into nonhospital settings to gain community-based experiences. However, other, perhaps greater, financial incentives— such as retaining the (often lower cost) clinical labor that residents provide—continue to override this objective.

Impacts of Hospital Focus on Residency Experience

Inpatient hospital experience provides residents with important exposure to serious illnesses, but it must be balanced with sufficient experience in nonhospital and community-based settings. For most specialties, learning how to successfully manage a patient's medical conditions outside the hospital is important for patient health, patient comfort, and Medicare spending. Yet, inherent financial incentives and payment regulations discourage teaching hospitals from establishing strong offsite affiliations and, in limiting residents' experiences, may ultimately affect residents' specialty and setting choice for their future medical practice. The Commission has raised concerns about the decline in the number of U.S. medical school graduates selecting primary care and geriatrics, and the growth in the number of internal medicine physicians deciding to subspecialize or become hospitalists. These trends likely contribute to a reduction in the number of physicians who continue to treat their patients when they enter nursing homes (Levy et al. 2005).

While accreditation organizations require at least some education and training in ambulatory care settings for many specialties, Medicare's subsidies for graduate medical education place no requirements on nonhospital experience. In the case of internal medicine, for example, ACGME requires that at least one-third of internal medicine residents' time must be in ambulatory sites. In many cases, residency programs fulfill this ambulatory requirement by rotating the residents to the teaching hospitals' own outpatient departments, clinics, and physician offices. These ambulatory rotations, which occur in hospital-owned facilities, do not place hospitals' graduate medical education payments at risk. However, the teaching hospitals' loss of residency time and labor remains a factor, potentially prompting the ambulatory care requirements instituted by accrediting organizations and specialty boards.

Work for Future Exploration

Medical education plays a key role in shaping new physicians' attitudes and skills with respect to health care delivery reforms. Accordingly, the Commission looks forward to more detailed discussions about possible reforms to the medical education process. In addition to further examination of ways to encourage more educational experience in nonhospital settings, we will focus our future analysis on three main areas, as outlined below.

Linking Medical Education Incentives with Delivery System Reforms

Linking Medicare's medical education subsidies to specific delivery system reforms could improve residents' education and training. This strategy is based on the premise that residents and other health professionals will be more likely to learn "best practices" when they are learning within a delivery system that is integrated, coordinated, high quality, and focused on the efficient provision of care. Medical education incentives could include, for example, higher subsidies to entities with infrastructure that facilitates high-quality efficient care, such as integrated care and communication among providers across different types of health care settings. The main objective in linking medical education subsidies to delivery system reforms would be to shift more payments to the hospitals and residency programs that emphasize superior quality and judicious resource use and away from those structured more heavily on long-established, volume-based incentives.

Another focus could be on selected payment reforms that concentrate on managing the quality and efficiency of care across providers and settings. For example, hospitals and physician offices that accept bundled payments for all Part A and Part B services in a given episode of care could receive higher medical education subsidies. Curricula that specialize in delivery system reforms, such as care-coordination techniques and cost awareness, could also be recognized. Also, because faculty expertise is an influential factor in residency program curricula, efforts to encourage programs and institutions to educate existing core faculty—as well as recruit other faculty with selected expertise in such topics as quality measurement and improvement—could be effective. Other curricular incentives could include basic instruction in geriatric care across all specialties. The Commission recognizes, however, that resident education and interest are strongly influenced by the content and format of board certification exams.

Structuring Medical Education Subsidies to Produce the Professionals We Need

The Commission will also examine ways for medical education subsidies to help generate a balance of advanced health care professionals that efficiently meets the needs of Medicare patients and the U.S. population at large. Among physicians, nurses, and physician assistants, it is important to achieve the right share of generalists and subspecialists. Although the exact balance may evolve over time, the Commission is particularly concerned about access to health professionals who provide primary care, such as those focusing on family, internal, geriatric, and pediatric medicine. These professionals and other generalists, such as general surgeons, are essential for a well-functioning health care delivery system. Thus, if medical education subsidies were to more strongly favor programs that educate and train generalists, then teaching institutions (e.g., teaching hospitals) may be more inclined to invest in these programs. Nevertheless, the influence of reimbursement differentials for primary care and procedural services and widely known income disparities between these specialties present a major hurdle for recruiting residents into generalist specialties.

We will also explore other ways to recruit health professionals, including physicians, nurse practicioners, and physician assistants, who can most effectively help reform our health care delivery system. For example, loan forgiveness policies may help to attract students from diverse economic, ethnic, and geographic backgrounds. Increased support for advanced nursing education and training programs could focus attention on these key team members for improving the coordination of care. Considering Medicare's subsidy of approximately $100,000 per resident per year, Medicare could require practicing physicians to conduct some minimal public service in exchange for this support. For example, they could be required to provide occasional on-call services at hospitals or in other settings after their residency. Such a requirement would necessitate long-term contractual agreements from the resident, and some contend that this process could be complicated and that physicians should not be expected to donate their time simply because the government made some investments on their behalf. Having an adequate panel of local physicians on call is a crucial component of the nation's access to health care, yet, in recent years, fewer physicians are agreeing to take call (CHCF 2005).

Enlisting Other Payers to Contribute Explicitly to Medical Education

Currently Medicare, Medicaid, and other federal programs are the largest funders of graduate medical education. Although a small number of states require private insurers to contribute toward this endeavor, most do not. Some private insurers report that they support graduate medical education indirectly through higher patient care payments to teaching-affiliated health care providers. Considering the shared, societal benefits of high-quality medical education, the Commission will analyze options for all insurers to contribute explicitly to the costs of educating our nation's medical professionals.

With additional sources of funding for medical education, several researchers have discussed the role of an independent board in making decisions about allocating medical education subsidies (COGME 2007, IOM 1997, Pew Center for Health Professions 1998, Whitcomb 2007). A goal for such a board would be to ensure the equitable and efficient distribution of funds to appropriate entities that provide medical education and training across all ages. For graduate medical education, these entities could include teaching hospitals, nonhospital settings, and even residency programs. Goals guiding the distribution of these funds could stem from the objectives described previously, such as delivery system reforms and adjusting the balance of health care professionals to ensure adequate access to primary care.

REFERENCES

[1] Accreditation Council for Graduate Medical Education. (2008). *Educating physicians for the 21st century.* Chicago: ACGME. http://www.acgme.org/Outcome/.

[2] American Academy of Family Physicians. (2009). *Transforming graduate medical education.* Policy document. Washington, DC: AAFP. http://www.aafp.org/online/etc/medialib/aafp_org/documents/policy/fed/background/gme03 1009. Par. 0001. File. tmp/ TransformingGME03 1009.pdf.

[3] American Association of Colleges of Osteopathic Medicine. (2009). *2009 annual statistical report on osteopathic medical education. Chevy Chase*, MD: AACOM.

[4] American Board of Medical Specialties. (2009). *How a physician becomes board certified.* Evanston, IL: ABMS. http://www.abms. org/ Who_ We_ Help/ Consumers/ process.aspx.

[5] American Medical Association. (2008). *State medical licensure requirements and statistics, 2008*. Chicago: AMA.

[6] Association of American Medical Colleges. (2009). *Getting into medical school.* Washington, DC: AAMC. http://www.aamc.org/ students/considering/gettingin.htm.

[7] Association of American Medical Colleges. (2008a). *Data warehouse: Applicant and matriculant file as of 10/10/2008.* Washington, DC: AAMC. http://www.aamc.org/data/facts.

[8] Association of American Medical Colleges. (2008b). *Diversity of U.S. medical students by parental income*. Analysis in brief, *vol. 8*, no. 1. Washington, DC: AAMC.

[9] Association of American Medical Colleges. (2008c). *Medical student education: Costs, debt, and loan repayment facts.* Washington, DC: AAMC.

[10] Association of American Medical Colleges. (2008d). Medicare DGME and IME payments: Counting resident time in didactic and research activities. *Presentation to MedPAC staff.*

[11] Babineau, T. J., Becker, J. & Gibbons, G., et al. (2004). The cost of operative training for surgical residents. *Archives of Surgery*, *139*, no. 4, 366-369.

[12] Berwick, D. M. (1996). A primer on leading the improvement of systems. *British Medical Journal*, *312*, 6 19-22.

[13] Blue Ridge Academic Health Group. (2003). *Reforming medical education: Urgent priority for the academic health center in the new century*. Report 7. Athens, GA: Emory University.

[14] Blumenthal, D. (2002). *Training tomorrow's doctors: The medical education mission of academic health centers*. New York: Commonwealth Fund.

[15] Blumenthal, D., Gokhale, J., Campbell, E. & Weissman. J. (2001). Preparedness for clinical practice. *Journal of the American Medical Association*, *286*, no. 9, 1027-1034.

[16] Brooks, R. G., Walsh, M., Mardon, R. E., et al. (2002). The roles of nature and nurture in the recruitment and retention of primary care

physicians in rural areas: A review of the literature. *Academic Medicine, 77*, 790-798.

[17] Brotherton, S. E. & Etzel, S. I. (2008). Graduate medical education, 2007-2008. *Journal of the American Medical Association, 300*, no. 10 (September 10), 1228-1243.

[18] California HealthCare Foundation. (2005). *On-call physicians at California emergency departments: Problems and potential solutions.* Issue brief. Oakland: CHCF.

[19] Cordasco, K., Horta, M., Lurie, N., et al. (2009). *How are residency programs preparing our 21st century internists? A review of internal medicine residency programs' teaching on selected topics*. Santa Monica, CA: RAND Corporation. Contractor report prepared for MedPAC.

[20] Council on Graduate Medical Education. (2007). *COGME 19th report: Enhancing flexibility in graduate medical education.* Washington, DC: COGME.

[21] Council on Graduate Medical Education. (1999). *COGME 13th report: Physician education for a changing health care environment.* Washington, DC: COGME.

[22] Federation of State Medical Boards. 2009. *Maintenance of licensure, frequently asked questions.* Dallas, TX: FSMB. http:// www.fsmb.o rg/m_mol_faqs.html.

[23] Fordyce, M., Chen, F., Doescher, M. & Hart. L. (2007). *2005 Physician supply and distribution in rural areas of the United States.* University of Washington Rural Health Research Center. Report 116. Prepared for The Federal Office of Rural Health Policy, Health Resources and Services Administration, Department of Health and Human Services.

[24] Freeman, E. & Lischka, T. (2009). Osteopathic graduate medical education. *Journal of the American Osteopathic Association, 109*, no. 3, 135-145.

[25] Gorman, P. J., Meier, A. H., Rawn, C., et al. (2000). The future of medical education is no longer blood and guts, it is bites and bytes. *American Journal of Surgery, 180*, no. 5, 353-356.

[26] Grumbach, K. & Mendoza, R. (2008). Disparities in human resources: Addressing the lack of diversity in the health professions. *Health Affairs, 27*, no. 2, 413-422.

[27] Health Resources and Services Administration. (2006). *The rationale for diversity in the health professions: A review of the evidence*. Rockville, MD, HRSA. October. ftp://ftp.hrsa.gov/bhpr/ workforce/diversity.pdf.

[28] Holmboe, E. S., Bowen, J. L., Green, M., et al. (2005). Reforming internal medicine residency training. *Journal of General Internal Medicine*, *20*, no. 12, 1165-1172.

[29] Institute of Medicine. (2008). *Retooling for an aging America: Building the health care workforce.* Washington, DC: National Academy Press.

[30] Institute of Medicine. (2004a). *In the nation's compelling interest: Ensuring diversity in the health care workforce.* Washington, DC: National Academy Press.

[31] Institute of Medicine. (2004b). *Academic health centers: Leading change in the 21st century*. Washington, DC: National Academy Press.

[32] Institute of Medicine. (2003). *Health professions education: A bridge to quality*. Washington, DC: National Academy Press.

[33] Institute of Medicine. (1997). *On implementing a national graduate medical education trust fund*. Washington, DC: National Academy Press.

[34] Johnson, T., Shah, M., Rechner, J., et al. (2008). Evaluating the effect of resident involvement on physician productivity in an academic general internal medicine practice. *Academic Medicine*, *83*, no. 7 (July), 670-674.

[35] Komaromy, M., Grumbach, K., Drake, M., et al. (1996). The role of black and Hispanic physicians in providing health care for underserved populations. *New England Journal of Medicine*, *334*, no. 20, 1305-13 10.

[36] Lave, Judith, R. (1985). *The Medicare adjustment for the indirect cost of medical education: Historical developments and current status.* Washington, DC: AAMC.

[37] Levy, C., Epstein, A., Landry, L., et al. (2005). *Literature review and synthesis of physician practices in nursing homes*. Denver: University of Colorado, Health Sciences Center. Report prepared under contract to ASPE/HHA.

[38] Ludmerer, K. & Johns, M. (2005). Reforming graduate medical education. *Journal of the American Medical Association*, *294*, no. 9, 1083-1087.

[39] Medicare Payment Advisory Commission. (2008). *Report to the Congress: Reforming the delivery system.* Washington, DC: MedPAC.

[40] Medicare Payment Advisory Commission, (2007). *Report to the Congress: Medicare payment policy*. Washington, DC: MedPAC.

[41] Medicare Payment Advisory Commission. (2005). *Report to the Congress: Medicare payment policy*. Washington, DC: MedPAC.

[42] Mertz, E. A. & Grumbach, K. (2001). Identifying communities with low dentist supply in California. *Journal of Public Health Dentistry*, *61*, no. 3, 172-177.

[43] Meyers, F., Weinberger, S., Fitzgibbons, J., et al. (2007). Redesigning residency training in internal medicine: The consensus report of the alliance for academic internal medicine education redesign task force. *Academic Medicine*, *82*, 1211-1219.

[44] Moy, E. & Bartman, B. A. (1995). Physician race and care of minority and medically indigent patients. *Journal of the American Medical Association*, *273*, no. 19, 1515-1520.

[45] Mullan, F. (2009). Workforce issues in health care reform: Assessing the present and preparing for the future. *Testimony before the Senate Finance Committee*. March 12.

[46] Nasca, Thomas. (2008). Statement at MedPAC meeting. October 2.

[47] Ogrine, G., L. Headrick, A., Mutha, S., et al. (2003). A framework for teaching medical students and residents about practice based learning and improvement, synthesized from a literature review. *Academic Medicine*, *78*, no. 7, 748-756.

[48] Peters, A., Clark-Chiarelli, N. & Block, S. (1999). Comparison of osteopathic and allopathic medical schools' support for primary care. *Journal of General Internal Medicine*, *14*, no. 12, 730-739.

[49] Pew Center for Health Professions. (1998). *Beyond the Balanced Budget Act of 1997, Strengthening federal GME policy.* San Francisco: Pew Center for Health Professions. Executive summary of the full report.

[50] Rich, E. C., Liebow, M., Srinivasan, M., et al. (2002). Medicare financing of graduate medical education: Intractable problems, elusive solutions. *Journal of General Internal Medicine*, *12*, 283-292.

[51] Salsberg, E., Rockey, P. H., Rivers, K. L., et al. (2008). US residency training before and after the 1997 Balanced Budget Act. *Journal of the American Medical Association*, *300*, no. 10, 1174-1180.

[52] Shortell, S. M., Gillies, R. R. & Anderson, D. A. (2000). *Remaking health care in America*. 2nd ed. San Francisco: JosseyBass.

[53] Steinbrook, R. (2008). Medical student debt—is there a limit? *New England Journal of Medicine*, *359*, 2629-2632.

[54] Stewart, M., Meredith, L., Brown, J. B., et al. (2000). The influence of older patient-physician communication on health and health- related outcomes. *Clinics in Geriatric Medicine*, *16*, no. 1, 25-36.

[55] U.S. House. (1965). 89th Cong., 1st sess. *32*, H.R. 213.

[56] U.S. Senate. (1965). 89th Cong., 1st sess. *36*, S.R. 404, pt. 1.

[57] Weinberger, S. E., Smith, L. G., Collier, V. U., et al. (2006). Redesigning training for internal medicine. *Annals of Internal Medicine, 144*, 927-932.

[58] White, K. L., Williams, F. & Greenberg, B. G. (1961). The ecology of medical care. *New England Journal of Medicine*, 265 (November 2), 885-892.

[59] Wickstrom, G., Kolar, M., Keyserling, C., et al. (2000). Confidence of graduating internal medicine residents to perform ambulatory procedures. *Journal of General Internal Medicine, 15*, 36 1-365.

[60] Wiest, F., Ferris, T., Gokhale, M., et al. (2002). Preparedness of internal medicine and family practice residents for treating common conditions. *Journal of the American Medical Association, 288*, 2609-26 14.

[61] Wolff, J. L., Starfield, B. & Anderson, G. (2002). Prevalence, expenditures and complications of multiple chronic conditions in the elderly. *Archives of Internal Medicine, 162*, 2269-2276.

[62] Wynn, B., Guarino, C., Morse, L., et al. (2006). *Alternative ways of financing graduate medical education*. RAND working paper. Santa Monica, CA: RAND Corporation. May.

End Notes

[1] There were also 11,742 applicants for 4,389 positions in osteopathic medical schools in 2008. As there is some overlap between the applicant pools, the total number of unique applicants to allopathic and osteopathic medical schools combined cannot be determined.

[2] Osteopathic residency programs have their own match structured in a similar fashion to the NRMP match.

[3] The binding commitment is for one year. Residents can choose to change programs after the first year of training, if they find a program willing to accept them.

[4] Colorado, Indiana, New York, South Dakota, and Vermont have no minimum CME requirements.

[5] Illinois, Kansas, Maine, Massachusetts, Michigan, New Hampshire, New Jersey, North Carolina, Ohio, Pennsylvania, and Washington require an average of 50 credit hours.

[6] The American Board of Medical Specialties on March 16, 2009, adopted a new set of standards for the MOC program that the individual specialty boards will incorporate into their MOC programs from 2010 to 2012. These new standards include self-assessment requirements, evidence of participation in practice-based assessment and quality improvement, patient safety assessment, and evaluation of communication assessment skills.

[7] In addition to the allopathic and osteopathic accreditation, dental and podiatry programs accredited by their respective accrediting bodies also qualify.

[8] This support totals about $300 million and is limited to programs sponsored by the hospital, mostly diploma programs, which have been replaced by associate and baccalaureate programs sponsored by community colleges and universities, which are ineligible for Medicare support, even though some training may take place in the hospital. Title VII,

administered through the Health Resources and Services Administration, also provides funding for nurse education.

[9] Approximately 19,000 of these residents were counted as half an FTE for direct GME payments because the trainees were in either a subspecialty fellowship—having completed their initial residency—or training beyond the minimum required for initial board certification in a specialty.

[10] With the total Medicare-supported residents and the 8,000 additional residents, in 2006 there were about 97,800 FTE residents training in Medicare-supported hospitals (91,800 in short-stay acute care hospitals). A little more than 7,000 residents were in non-inpatient prospective payment system hospitals (e.g., cancer hospitals, children's hospitals).

[11] Exceptions may apply for new programs established in rural hospitals, hospitals that had no residents in the base period, and urban hospitals with a new separately accredited rural training track.

[12] Provided they are fully licensed, residents may bill Medicare for (moonlighting) services they provide that are not considered part of their residency training experience.

[13] There is also an IME adjustment that is made to capital payment rates that is based on a different formula. Capital IME payments, which totaled about $360 million in 2007, are scheduled to be eliminated by the Secretary in 2010. The inpatient rehabilitation facility prospective payment system (PPS), long-term care hospital PPS, and psychiatric hospital PPS also include an IME adjustment based on their own payment formulas.

[14] The study showed that physician productivity, as measured by relative value unit output, declined when residents were present in an internal medicine practice. Relative value unit output per hour declined by 0.8 when physicians were working with first- and second-year residents and by 0.5 when working with third-year residents.

[15] See, for example, Blue Ridge Academic Health Group 2003, Blumenthal 2002, COGME 2007, Holmboe et al. 2005, IOM 2008, IOM 2003, Ludmerer and Johns 2005, Meyers et al. 2007, Mullan 2009, Weinberger et al. 2006.

[16] In comparison with the universe of U.S. internal medicine residency programs, the RAND researchers found that the randomly selected sample was representative on the following characteristics: number of residents, type of hospital (university, community, municipal), geographic region, and type of program accreditation (allopathic, osteopathic). Programs that had *both* allopathic and osteopathic accreditation were slightly oversampled.

[17] In preliminary research on medical school curriculum, we found that fewer than 10 percent of medical school programs include instruction on health care costs and spending as a requirement or objective in the curriculum.

[18] Beginning July 2003, the ACGME limited residents' duty hours to an 80-hour work week, averaged over 4 weeks. In December 2008, the IOM recommended further specifications on the need for a 5-hour sleep period.

[19] The hospital must incur at least 90 percent of the total of all the nonhospitals' associated training costs. CMS does not consider resident salaries and fringe benefits to equal "all or substantially all of the costs of the training program in the nonhospital setting." Prior to 1998, Medicare accepted resident salaries and fringe benefits as meeting this requirement in full.

[20] Effective July 1, 2007, in determining the teaching physician supervisory cost, hospitals may also use national average salary data in place of actual teaching physician salary information and may also use a proxy percentage representing the amount of time the teaching physician spends supervising the residents.

[21] The exceptions are Federally Qualified Health Centers, Rural Health Clinics, and Medicare+Choice organizations. These entities became eligible to receive direct GME and IME from Medicare through the Balanced Budget Act of 1997.

In: Graduate Medical Education Issues
Editor: Caroline I. Hansen et al.
ISBN: 978-1-61122-902-8

Chapter 3

GRADUATE MEDICAL EDUCATION FINANCING: FOCUSING ON EDUCATIONAL PRIORITIES

MedPac

RECOMMENDATIONS

4.1. The Congress should authorize the Secretary to change Medicare's funding of graduate medical education (GME) to support the workforce skills needed in a delivery system that reduces cost growth while maintaining or improving quality.

- The Secretary should establish the standards for distributing funds after consultation with representatives that include accrediting organizations, training programs, health care organizations, health care purchasers, patients, and consumers.
- The standards established by the Secretary should, in particular, specify ambitious goals for practice-based learning and improvement, interpersonal and communication skills, professionalism, and systems-based practice, including integration of community-based care with hospital care.
- Performance-based GME funding under the new system should be allocated to an institution sponsoring GME programs only if that

institution met the new standards established by the Secretary, and the level of funding would be tied to the institution's performance on the standards.

The indirect medical education (IME) payments above the empirically justified amount should be removed from the IME adjustment and that sum would be used to fund the new performance-based GME program. To allow time for the development of standards, the new performance-based GME program should begin in three years (October 2013).

4.2. The Secretary should annually publish a report that shows Medicare medical education payments received by each hospital and each hospital's associated costs. This report should be publicly accessible and clearly identify each hospital, the direct and indirect medical education payments received, the number of residents and other health professionals that Medicare supports, and Medicare's share of teaching costs incurred.

4.3. The Secretary should conduct workforce analysis to determine the number of residency positions needed in the United States in total and by specialty. In addition, analysis should examine and consider the optimal level and mix of other health professionals. This work should be based on the workforce requirements of health care delivery systems that provide high-quality, high-value, and affordable care.

4.4. The Secretary should report to the Congress on how residency programs affect the financial performance of sponsoring institutions and whether residency programs in all specialties should be supported equally.

4.5. The Secretary should study strategies for increasing the diversity of our health professional workforce (e.g., increasing the shares from underrepresented rural, lower income, and minority communities) and report on what strategies are most effective to achieve this pipeline goal.

SUMMARY

Our nation's system of medical education and graduate training produces superbly skilled clinicians while contributing to stunning advances in medical science. Yet, it is not aligned with the delivery system reforms essential for increasing the value of health care in the United States. Research discussed in our June 2009 report, for example, found that internal medicine residency programs had limited focus on skills such as quality measurement and improvement, evidence-based medicine, multidisciplinary teamwork, care coordination across settings, and health information technology. These skills are important for producing the health professionals we need for a high-performance delivery system—one that provides high quality, high value, and efficiently delivered services.

Medicare is the single largest payer of graduate medical education (GME)— $9.5 billion in 2009—but requires minimal accountability from its recipients for achieving education and training goals. Approximately $3 billion of Medicare's payments is intended to support Medicare's share of the direct costs of running GME programs. The other $6.5 billion is intended to support Medicare's share of the indirect clinical costs associated with the presence of GME. Commission analysis has shown that this amount is $3.5 billion higher than the empirically calculated indirect clinical costs associated with teaching (Medicare Payment Advisory Commission 2010).

This chapter presents the Commissions' summary assessment of gaps in the current GME system—with particular attention to financing issues—and makes a set of recommendations to address some of the identified concerns. Two principles underlying these recommendations are: the need to decouple Medicare's GME payments from fee-for-service (FFS) payment systems, and the need to ensure that resources for GME are devoted to meeting educational standards and outcomes that can improve the value of our health care delivery system. We also discuss the importance of understanding workforce requirements for improved health care delivery in the 21st century.

Commission's Summary Assessment of the GME System

Despite the tremendous advances that our GME system has brought to modern health care, the Commission finds it is not consistently producing physicians and other health professionals who can become leaders in reforming our delivery system to substantially improve its quality and value. Two specific areas of concern are workforce mix—including trends in specialization and limited socioeconomic diversity—and education and training in skills needed for improving the value of our health care delivery system—including evidence-based medicine, team-based care, care coordination, and shared decision making.

We cannot accomplish delivery system reform without simultaneously ensuring that the providers we need have the skills necessary to integrate care across settings, improve quality, and use resources efficiently. In a recent *New England Journal of Medicine* article, prominent physicians assert that not only do residents need to learn relatively new skills, they need to develop a new perspective on what it means to be a "good doctor"—shifting emphasis, for example, from independent and autonomous practice to more patient-centered, team-based care (Swensen et al. 2010).

Our GME system is influenced not only by how Medicare subsidizes it but also by how Medicare and other insurers pay for health care services. FFS payment systems reward volume without regard to quality and their levels of payment for physician services tend to reward performing procedures over patient evaluation, management, and care coordination. These payment signals likely affect not only physician career choices but also institutional decisions about which residency programs to offer.

Commission Recommendations to Address Gaps in the GME System

First, the Commission recommends increasing accountability for Medicare's GME payments. We recommend establishing a performance-based incentive program with payments to institutions contingent on reaching desired educational outcomes and standards. Eligible institutions would include teaching hospitals, medical schools, and other entities that may sponsor residency programs. In determining the criteria for evaluating performance under this program, the Secretary of Health and Human Services would consult with organizations and individuals with the necessary expertise and perspectives—specifically, representatives from organizations such as program accrediting bodies, certifying boards, training programs, health care organizations, health care purchasers, and patient and consumer groups. From these deliberations, the Secretary would develop a GME payment system that fosters greater accountability for Medicare's GME dollars and rewards education and training that will improve the value of our health care delivery system. Although accrediting standards for residency programs are moving in this direction, the Commission recommends that Medicare institute financial incentives to accelerate these efforts.

Funding for this initiative should come from reducing Medicare's indirect medical education (IME) payments to eliminate the amount currently paid above empirically justified IME costs. Although some could assert that this amount should not be expended at all, the Commission determined that Medicare should use this amount to fund incentive payments to institutions meeting specified educational standards. Only those institutions meeting these educational standards specified by the Secretary should be eligible for such incentive payments; conceivably, therefore, all, some, or none of this amount could be distributed, depending on performance. Future assessment of the GME payment system might consider making even larger portions of Medicare's GME payments contingent on performance.

Second, the Commission recommends making information about Medicare's payments and teaching costs available to the public to foster greater accountability for educational activities within the GME community. To encourage collaboration between educators and institutions on residency program funding decisions, Medicare should make information about GME payments and costs more accessible. Although interpreting reported cost data may require some caveats, the transparency of this payment and cost information will recognize Medicare's significant investment in residency (and some nursing) training and education.

The final three recommendations in this chapter call for studies to examine specific aspects of health workforce training. Currently, Medicare's payments for GME generally subsidize the specialty choices of both teaching hospitals (in their program offerings) and residents (in their career choices). The resulting physician mix of specialties is unlikely to ensure that the nation has an efficient supply of health professionals for well-functioning delivery systems, as evidenced by falling shares of physicians practicing primary care after their residencies. The Commission recommends that a rigorous, independent analysis of our health care workforce be conducted regularly. This analysis should be driven by the requirements of a high-value, affordable health care delivery system. Analyses that simply extrapolate demand projections based on current patterns of care could compromise the nation's chances of fostering high-value health care systems. An improved delivery system will influence the total number of physicians and the mix of professionals needed in our health workforce. Consequently, any decisions about Medicare's funding of new residency positions should await the results of such a study.

Also in question is the optimal level of Medicare GME payments by resident specialty type. Institutional costs and benefits of supporting residency programs are likely to vary significantly by specialty. For example, some specialties may require greater supervision costs, while others may attract higher volumes of more profitable services to the institution. There is little research on these differences. To learn how Medicare could adjust its subsidies for residency programs to make them more economically efficient, a specialty-specific analysis of net institutional costs and benefits would be useful.

A third workforce goal that deserves concerted attention is to find the most effective strategies for increasing the diversity of our pipeline of health professionals (i.e., increasing the share of professionals from underrepresented racial and ethnic minorities, from lower income families, and from rural hometowns). Research has found that a diverse health care workforce is associated with better care quality and access for disadvantaged populations, greater patient choice and satisfaction, and better educational experience for students in health professions. A number of programs, administered by the Health Resources and Services Administration, are designed to address this goal. While research on several specific programs shows some positive impacts, comprehensive evaluation of these programs' longitudinal effectiveness is not well studied. Therefore, a study that outlines a strategy for achieving specific health care workforce-diversity goals is essential to optimize federal subsidies for this effort.

Over the last two years, as the Commission examined ways to improve graduate medical education (GME) financing, it became clear that delivery system reform cannot be accomplished without simultaneously ensuring that the physicians and other health professionals we need have the skills necessary to integrate care across settings, improve quality, and use resources efficiently. Although the nation's GME system produces superbly skilled clinicians and stunning advances in medical science, greater attention is needed to align its educational goals with the nation's delivery system needs. This chapter presents the Commission's assessment of problems in the GME system and offers a set of recommendations. Two principles underlying these recommendations are: the need to decouple Medicare's GME payments from fee-for-service (FFS) payment systems, and the need to ensure that resources for GME are devoted to meeting educational standards and outcomes that can improve the value of our health care delivery system. We also discuss the importance of understanding and meeting health care workforce goals for the 21st century.

Commission's Summary Assessment of the GME System

Our nation's system of GME is, in some respects, the best in the world: U.S. teaching hospitals produce thousands of new physicians each year—physicians who are superbly skilled and able to apply cutting-edge technology and techniques to aid severely ill or injured patients. Teaching hospitals often serve as linchpins of their local health care systems, and many contribute to stunning advances in medical science.

The GME system is not, however, consistently producing the physicians and other health professionals needed for a 21st century health care delivery system, one focused on high-quality, high-value, and affordable care. That is not just our assessment but also the assessment of some active participants in GME as well as many health care delivery organizations, insurers, corporate purchasers, and organizations representing patients and consumers (Blumenthal 2002, Council on Graduate Medical Education 2007b, Holmboe et al. 2005, Institute of Medicine 2008, Ludmerer and Johns 2005, Meyers et al. 2007, Mullan 2009, Swensen et al. 2010).

Gaps in the Current GME System

We find gaps in the mix of physicians being produced (including their specialty, their geographic distribution, and their socioeconomic diversity) and in the content of their education and training. (In addition, there are distinct, but complementary, problems in the education and training of other health professionals, which are critical as well. However, this chapter focuses principally on the training of physicians, as does Medicare's GME funding.)

Physician mix

The specialty mix of physicians coming through the GME pipeline is not well matched to the needs of an efficient, high-quality, high-value delivery system. As discussed in our June 2009 report, a reformed delivery system that focuses on effective chronic care and keeping patients from needing to be hospitalized will require primary care physicians who can function with other health care professionals and specialists as part of a patient's health care team. These primary care providers are essential to a well-functioning delivery system, yet the mix of specialists and primary care graduates from residency programs has been tilting more toward specialists (American College of Physicians 2006, Colwill et al. 2008). Specifically, the proportion of third-year internal medicine residents becoming generalists is declining because a growing share is choosing to subspecialize or become hospitalists after residency (Bodenheimer 2006).[1]

In addition, there is insufficient socioeconomic diversity among physicians entering the pipeline, and too few are drawn from rural areas and inner cities, which may mean a reduced propensity to practice in these often underserved areas. Studies show that residents tend to select practice locations that are similar to where they grew up and where they trained (Brooks et al. 2002, Phillips et al. 2009). Yet, medical schools and residency programs are concentrated in certain areas of the country and draw students from families with considerably higher incomes than the population at large has (Association of American Medical Colleges 2008). Socioeconomic diversity in the physician workforce is crucial for improving patient access to culturally responsive care. In addition to programs sponsored by the Health Resources and Services Administration (HRSA), efforts to increase physician workforce diversity have been undertaken by private foundations and other organizations such as the Association of American Medical Colleges, but diversity is still insufficient, suggesting that we need to examine the effectiveness of current strategies.

Additionally, prudent workforce strategies need to address other health professionals, such as nurse practitioners and physician assistants, who provide essential patient care and enhance the effectiveness and efficiency of physician time and expertise.

Content and outcomes of physician training

The GME system should embrace a more systematic effort to instill the skills and perspectives needed to accelerate the development of a high-quality, high-value, and efficient delivery system, including (but not limited to) evidence- based medicine, team-based care, care coordination, and shared decision making. A recent article authored by numerous well-regarded physicians asserts that not only do residents need to learn relatively new skills, they also need to develop a new perspective on what it means to be a "good doctor"—shifting emphasis, for example, from independent and autonomous practice, to more patient- centered, team-based care (Swensen et al. 2010).

A reformed delivery system will require health care professionals trained to provide coordinated care across institutional boundaries and trained in the skills required to promote patient safety and quality. Yet, studies show that this kind of training is not routinely provided in residency programs today (Cordasco et al. 2009, Council on Graduate Medical Education 2007a, Council on Graduate Medical Education 2007b, Lucien Leape Institute 2010, Medicare Payment Advisory Commission 2009). These findings suggest that although the Accreditation Coucil for Graduate Medical Education (ACGME) has begun instituting outcome-based standards for some of these newer skills and competencies, progress on them has been slow. Some of these shortfalls are compounded by a GME system focused too heavily on inpatient care. Although experience in caring for hospital inpatients is an indispensable part of a physician's education, greater focus on providing ambulatory care for chronically ill patients with complex health care needs is essential for preventing avoidable hospitalizations and improving overall care delivery.

Payers' role in fostering gaps in GME system

The GME system is not solely responsible for these gaps and problems. Medicare has played a large role in shaping— some would say distorting—the GME system. GME is influenced not only by how Medicare subsidizes it but also by how Medicare pays for health care services. In making decisions about their clinical and training priorities, teaching hospitals likely consider financial signals from Medicare about what types of care are most valued. Those signals are embedded in the methods used to pay for services and the relative rates paid for different services. For example, Medicare's FFS payment system rewards volume without regard to quality. At the same time, the physician payment system has tended to reward procedural over cognitive care. While the Congress and CMS have increased payments for some cognitive services, the rewards for high volumes of lucrative procedures cannot help but influence hospitals' choices of which specialty residency programs to support and the programs' relative sizes.

Payment levels are also an important influence—although not the only influence—on the specialty preferences of physicians in training. Although lifestyle factors and the nature of the clinical and administrative work affect career choices, residents—many of whom face large debt levels for their education—reasonably look at future earnings prospects when choosing a specialty. Medicare payment rates can influence that choice. The payment methods used by other insurers, which are often based on Medicare's system, intensify these signals.

Medicare's Role in GME Reform

Aside from changes in the way Medicare pays for services, Medicare can modify its GME financing structure to support and accelerate delivery system reforms. Currently, some GME payments are calculated as a percentage add-on to inpatient hospital admissions and others are calculated based on Medicare's share of patient days; neither of these methods is an effective means for encouraging hospitals to foster ideal educational programs and environments. Thus, where possible, Medicare's subsidies for GME should be decoupled from its payment for services and instead directed toward educational goals (see the text box for a description of Medicare's current GME payments in more detail).

Delivery system reform cannot be accomplished without simultaneously ensuring that the physicians and health care professionals we need across this country have the skills necessary to integrate care across settings, improve quality, and use resources efficiently. The Commission considered whether federal subsidies for GME should be removed from Medicare and instead distributed through general revenues. Although a case could be made for this approach—considering that GME is thought by many to be a public good that benefits the nation as a whole— there were concerns with GME funding stability among other issues. On balance, the Commission determined that significant improvements can be accomplished through adjustments to current Medicare payment policies.

MEDICARE'S PAYMENTS FOR GRADUATE MEDICAL EDUCATION

Since its inception, Medicare has provided substantial support for graduate medical education (GME) in the United States. Its primary mechanism for these subsidies is through payments to teaching hospitals to support their higher patient care costs and physician residency programs. Medicare's GME payments for 2009 totaled an estimated $9.5 billion—averaging more than $100,000 per resident. These payments are divided into direct and indirect GME payments.

Direct GME (DGME) payments are intended to support the teaching aspects of residency programs, such as resident stipends and benefits, supervisory physician salaries, and administrative overhead expenses. DGME payments are based on a hospital-specific per resident payment amount that was determined in 1984, updated for inflation. This amount is applied to Medicare's share of the hospital's inpatient days (both fee-for-service and Medicare Advantage). Subspecialty fellowship positions are funded at half the amount of core-year residency positions. The total number of residents supported by Medicare is capped per hospital at 1996 levels. Medicare also provides some education funding to hospitals to support direct costs of hospital-based education and training programs for nursing and various allied health professions. Medicare's DGME payments totaled an estimated $3 billion in 2009.

Indirect medical education (IME) payments are designed to support the higher costs of patient care associated with teaching, such as residents' "learning by doing," greater use of emerging technologies, and patient severity. Based on a formula, IME payments are an adjustment—a percentage increase—to Medicare's inpatient payment rates and vary based on hospitals' "teaching intensity" (as measured by the ratio of residents to hospital beds). Therefore, hospitals' IME payments are tied to their Medicare inpatient volume and case mix as well as the size of their residency programs (subject to their resident cap number). Medicare makes separate adjustments for operating and capital payments. Hospitals also receive IME payments from Medicare for Medicare Advantage patients.

Medicare's IME payments totaled an estimated $6.5 billion in 2009, but repeated Commission analysis finds that only 40 percent to 45 percent of these payments can be analytically justified to cover the higher patient care costs of Medicare inpatients. In essence, the current adjustment is set at more than twice what can be empirically justified, resulting in an estimated $3.5 billion directed to teaching hospitals with little accountability for their use of these funds.

Federally qualified health centers, rural health clinics, and Medicare Advantage plans that sponsor residency training programs can also receive Medicare DGME payments. In the future, teaching health centers (established in the Patient Protection and Affordable Care Act of 2010 as community-based, ambulatory patient care centers that support primary care residency programs) will receive payments to support direct and indirect costs, but funding will be authorized in a manner similar to that for the Children's Hospital GME program (CHGME) and will not come from Medicare. The Health Services and Resources Administration manages the CHGME program and will manage the teaching health centers program.

Physician Mix

The single most important way Medicare can influence the mix of physicians being produced by the GME system is to reform how it pays for services. The Commission discussed the importance of promoting primary care and testing other payment models, such as medical homes, in its June 2008 report. The Congress and CMS have also taken steps toward these goals. If Medicare changes its signals about what care is valued, the GME system will likely respond.

Given the fiscal challenges confronting the federal government, current federal subsidies for physician and other health professional training should ideally be redesigned, not increased. If there is any increase in the number of residents Medicare supports, it should be founded on a careful analysis of future workforce needs that is driven by the needs of an efficient, high-quality, high-value system. An extrapolation of workforce needs based on current patterns of care would not just fail to meet the future needs of a high-quality, high-value, efficient delivery system, it could compromise the nation's chances of developing such a system by producing increasing numbers of providers who have a stake in the status quo.

Content and outcomes of physician training

Medicare should move toward a more accountable GME payment system that focuses on improving educational performance among institutions and residency programs. Such reforms likely will result in redistribution of current Medicare GME payments. Accordingly, changing how Medicare subsidizes GME should catalyze improvements in the content of GME instruction and resident experience. Although ACGME's outcome-based standards for residency programs are moving in this direction (as described later in this chapter) the Commission recommends that Medicare institute financial incentives to accelerate these efforts.

Medicare should not unilaterally presume to prescribe curricular content or teaching method. Any criteria for educational content should be the product of deliberation among parties with the necessary expertise and perspective, including accrediting organizations, certifying boards, government advisory bodies, teaching institutions, residency program directors, leading health care delivery systems, insurers, purchasers, and patients. Through ensuring that such deliberations proceed with the necessary speed and focus, Medicare can specify the results it expects from its substantial investment in GME and structure payment incentives that help align the educational process to those outcomes.

Role of other Federal Programs

Federal programs other than Medicare could also contribute to improving the output of the GME system as well as to the development of other important health professionals. Several HRSA programs are designed to attract individuals—particularly from minority, rural, and low-income comm.-unities—to health careers through a variety of incentives, ranging from early education (grade school) programs to loan repayment programs. HRSA programs are also focused on promoting primary care access, particularly in underserved areas, and enhancing the cultural competence of this workforce by funding opportunities for medical students and residents to train in diverse settings and locations. These programs have the potential to improve the mix of health professionals (through increases in socioeconomic diversity, rural access, and primary care providers) and should be subject to rigorous evaluation and improvement.

Second only to Medicare, Medicaid is another financer of GME. Because many states currently base their GME payments on Medicare's structure, changes in Medicare GME payment policies may also affect Medicaid policies. The Department of Veterans Affairs (VA) is also an active participant in GME, with more than one-third of residents rotating through VA facilities during their training. Research has shown that residents who rotate through the VA system gain delivery system skills, such as competencies in comprehensive health information technologies and multidisciplinary teamwork (Byrne et al. 2010, Congressional Budget Office 2007, Cordasco et al. 2009). Thus, the VA is likely to be an important partner in improving the GME system.

Commission Recommendations to Address Gaps in the GME System

In consideration of these identified concerns, the Commission makes a set of recommendations to address fundamental weaknesses in Medicare's system of GME subsidies. Two principles inherent in these recommendations are: the need to decouple Medicare's GME payments from FFS payment systems and the need to ensure that resources for GME are devoted to meeting educational standards and outcomes that can improve the value of our health care delivery system. The recommendations include linking GME payments to performance on educational standards and outcomes, increasing the transparency of and accountability for these payments, examining how best to assess health care workforce needs, assessing the impact of residency programs on hospitals' financial performance, and identifying strategies for increasing the diversity of the nation's physician workforce.

Link Payments to Performance to Meet Education and Training Goals for Delivery System Reform

Financial incentives that link GME payments to performance on educational standards and outcomes— such as resident competencies and adequate faculty support—can be important tools for encouraging more rigorous educational agendas among institutions and residency programs. Particular focus should be on skills essential for delivery system reform, such as quality measurement and improvement, evidence-based medicine, multidisciplinary teamwork, care coordination across settings, and health information technology. Although accreditation standards are moving in this direction, the Commission recommends that Medicare institute GME financing policies to accelerate these efforts. Funding for performance-based incentives should come from a significant reduction in IME payments.

Accelerate the Progress of Improving GME Outcomes

Currently, Medicare's only method for ensuring accountability for educational standards is its requirement that residents be in accredited residency programs. Most physician residency programs are accredited—by ACGME, the Commission on Osteopathic College Accreditation, or both.[2] These accrediting bodies are private, nonprofit councils that evaluate and accredit residency programs in the United States. In addition to Medicare financing, program accreditation is a requirement for other aspects of GME, including board certification and state licensure. It is rare for programs to lose their accreditation status.[3]

The ACGME recently transitioned to an outcome-based evaluation process for its residency programs. This initiative took an important step forward in defining core competencies not only in medical knowledge and patient care but also in skills that are consistent with those required to support health care delivery reform. These skills include practice-based learning and improvement, interpersonal and communication skills, professionalism, and systems-based practice.[4] They are described in further detail in the text box (pp. 112–113).

Many within the medical education community state that ACGME's Outcomes Project and evaluations are moving in the right direction (Chaudhry et al. 2008, Holmboe et al. 2006, Papadakis et al. 2008). However, studies show that progress toward these goals is slow. For example, examining 26 internal medicine residency programs (selected from a nationally representative sampling frame), RAND researchers found that, overall, internal medicine residency programs were not placing attention on formal instruction and experience in skills essential for delivery system reform—such as teamwork, quality measurement, and cost awareness (Cordasco et al. 2009, Medicare Payment Advisory Commission 2009). These researchers noted that overall programs' curricula on these topics fell far short of recommendations from the Institute of Medicine and other experts. A number of physicians in a recent article stated that a reformed delivery system will require physicians who are trained in relatively new skills that will enable them to provide more patient- centered, team-based care that is coordinated across institutional boundaries (Swensen et al. 2010). Reports from other experts have noted that training in these topics is not routinely provided in residency programs today (Council on Graduate Medical Education 2007a, Council on Graduate Medical Education 2007b, Lucien Leape Institute 2010).

Other educational efforts are beginning to address deficits

Several educators and specialty-based organizations have embarked on comprehensive projects to help medical schools and residency programs improve their teaching methods and curricula. For example, through its "Milestones Project" the American Board of Internal Medicine is aiming to teach educators successful methods for engaging residents in ACGME competencies and measuring their observable progress, but current Medicare payment policies do not provide incentives for these endeavors. Other specialties, such as general surgery, are engaged in similar milestones projects to facilitate outcome-based evaluations. Certifying boards are also influential in residency programs' curriculum development.[5]

An educational goal that is particularly pertinent to Medicare is the growing need for basic geriatric competency among almost all our physicians, as called for by many experts, clinicians, and researchers (Boult et al. 2010, Institute of Medicine 2008, Leipzig et al. 2009). While many specialties require some form of geriatric instruction for ACGME accreditation, and several organizations have collaborated to develop a set of geriatric competencies for all medical students and residents, Medicare's GME financing does not place any requirements on geriatric skills and experience.[6] Encouraging basic knowledge in geriatric care among graduating residents would have important benefits for elderly Medicare beneficiaries.

Particular focus needed to increase experience in nonhospital settings

Another concern about current residency education and training is its limited residency experience in nonhospital settings, as found in the previously mentioned RAND research. Hospital inpatient experience is a vital component of residency education to gain exposure to acute, serious illnesses, but it is equally essential for residents to have adequate time and experience outside the hospital in settings such as physician practices, nursing facilities, and nonhospital clinics. Benefits include greater experience with the clinical management of chronic conditions and exposure to the need for good care coordination across settings. Improving residents' comfort level with care in ambulatory settings could increase their desire to practice community-based care, particularly when their experiences in these nonhospital settings are positive. GME payment policies should create incentives for institutions and residency programs to maintain strong community-based, ambulatory rotations for their residents.[7] Recent legislative changes provide some Medicare payment flexibility to promote clinical nonhospital residency experience as described in the text box (p. 114).

The Accreditation Council for Graduate Medical Education (ACGME) Common Program Requirements: General Competencies

Approved by the ACGME board february 13, 2007

The residency program must integrate the following ACGME competencies into the curriculum:

Patient Care

Residents must be able to provide patient care that is compassionate, appropriate, and effective for the treatment of health problems and the promotion of health.

Medical Knowledge

Residents must demonstrate knowledge of established and evolving biomedical, clinical, epidemiological, and social–behavioral sciences as well as the application of this knowledge to patient care.

Practice-based Learning and Improvement

Residents must demonstrate the ability to investigate and evaluate their care of patients, to appraise and assimilate scientific evidence, and to continuously improve patient care based on constant self-evaluation and lifelong learning. Residents are expected to develop skills and habits to be able to meet the following goals:

- identify strengths, deficiencies, and limits in one's knowledge and expertise.
- set learning and improvement goals.
- identify and perform appropriate learning activities.
- systematically analyze practice using quality improvement methods, and implement changes with the goal of practice improvement.
- incorporate formative evaluation feedback into daily practice.
- locate, appraise, and assimilate evidence from scientific studies related to their patients' health problems.
- use information technology to optimize learning.
- participate in the education of patients, families, students, residents, and other health professionals.

Interpersonal and Communication Skills

Residents must demonstrate interpersonal and communication skills that result in the effective exchange of information and collaboration with patients, their families, and health professionals. Residents are expected to:

- communicate effectively with patients, families, and the public, as appropriate, across a broad range of socioeconomic and cultural backgrounds.
- communicate effectively with physicians, other health professionals, and health-related agencies.
- work effectively as a member or leader of a health care team or other professional group.
- act in a consultative role to other physicians and health professionals.
- maintain comprehensive, timely, and legible medical records, if applicable.

Professionalism

Residents must demonstrate a commitment to carrying out professional responsibilities and an adherence to ethical principles. Residents are expected to demonstrate:

- compassion, integrity, and respect for others;
- responsiveness to patient needs that supersedes self-interest;
- respect for patient privacy and autonomy;
- accountability to patients, society, and the profession; and
- sensitivity and responsiveness to a diverse patient population, including but not limited to diversity in gender, age, culture, race, religion, disabilities, and sexual orientation.

Systems-based Practice

Residents must demonstrate an awareness of and responsiveness to the larger context and system of health care as well as the ability to call effectively on other resources in the system to provide optimal health care. Residents are expected to:

- work effectively in various health care delivery settings and systems relevant to their clinical specialty.
- coordinate patient care within the health care system relevant to their clinical specialty.
- incorporate considerations of cost awareness and risk–benefit analysis in patient or population-based care as appropriate.

- advocate for quality patient care and optimal patient care systems.
- work in interprofessional teams to enhance patient safety and improve patient care quality.
- participate in identifying system errors and implementing potential systems solutions.

Increase accountability through performance- based payments

To create stronger incentives for providing residents with the education, training, and experiences necessary to achieve desired educational goals and outcomes, Medicare should create payment incentives based on institutional and program performance. The development of standards for measuring performance in topics essential for delivery system reform should be a collaborative process whereby the Secretary of Health and Human Services consults with representatives from organizations, such as program accrediting bodies, certifying boards, training programs, health care organizations, health care purchasers, and patient and consumer groups.

The standards established by the Secretary should specify ambitious goals for practice-based learning and improvement (including quality measurement), interpersonal and communication skills (including cultural sensitivity), professionalism (including patient-centered care), and systems-based practice (including integration of care across community- and hospital-based settings). Standards should address educational outcomes as well as clinical environments. These standards may vary depending on the types of institutions to which they apply, including hospitals, medical schools, and other entities that support residency programs. The topics of interest are also part of ACGME's current program evaluations as discussed earlier (text box, pp. 112–113); therefore, Medicare's assessment of residency programs and institutional performance would build on topics familiar to residency programs, teaching hospitals, and other affiliated institutions.

Recent Payment Changes Provide Payment Flexibility to Promote Clinical Nonhospital Residency Experience

The Patient Protection and Affordable Care Act of 2010 made three changes to Medicare payment policies to make it easier for residency time in certain nonhospital settings to be eligible for direct graduate medical education (DGME) payments and indirect medical education (IME) payments, starting July 1, 2010. First, supporting institutions (including hospitals that may share in supporting the costs of residents) will no longer need to cover more than the residents' stipends and benefits to qualify for DGME and IME when they rotate outside the hospital. (Previously, hospitals needed to pay the nonhospital sites for their supervision.) Second, for DGME payments, institutions will now be able to count the time residents spend on didactic and scholarly activities outside the hospital provided they are in clinical settings. (Previously, such didactic time could be counted only if it occurred in the hospital.) Third, for IME payments, hospitals will also now be able to count the time residents spend in non–patient care activities (except research not related to a particular patient) if they take place in the hospital, including provider-based hospital outpatient departments.

Although these provisions relax the nonhospital regulations, teaching hospitals have expressed concern that some administrative barriers will continue to exist. Resident time spent in didactic or scholarly activities in nonhospital settings will continue to be ineligible for IME payments. Time that residents spend in settings that are not primarily devoted to patient care—such as state public health departments, county jails, and medical schools—will continue to be ineligible for Medicare DGME and IME payments.

This new program will increase the accountability of Medicare subsidies for GME. Funding for the program should come from a substantial reduction in current IME payments. Repeated Commission analysis shows that Medicare's current IME payments—paid as add- ons to hospitals' case-based payments—are in excess of empirical costs (by an estimated $3.5 billion in 2009). Although some could assert that this amount should not be expended at all (and thus remain in the Medicare trust fund), the Commission determined that Medicare should use this amount to fund a new performance-based program.

As described above, this new program would establish payment incentives that reward institutions—including teaching hospitals, medical schools, and other entities that may support residency programs—which meet specified educational standards and outcomes. Only those institutions meeting these criteria should be eligible for such incentive payments; conceivably, therefore, all, some, or none of this amount could be distributed, based on program and institutional performance. Future assessment of the GME payment system might consider making even larger portions contingent on performance.

By rewarding successful teaching on topics such as quality measurement, teamwork, and cost awareness, Medicare would support efforts to produce a health care workforce with the skills needed for delivery system reform. Accordingly, institutions that offered greater support for educators' teaching time would likely experience better educational outcomes and thus could earn higher payments from Medicare. Additionally, standards for achieving higher payments could include hospitals' protection of faculty teaching time and investment in faculty expertise and development.

To allow adequate time for the development of educational standards and criteria, Medicare's new, more accountable payment approach should begin in three years—October 2013. This implementation date would also give hospitals and other qualified institutions some time to consider ways to improve their medical education programs and alter their operations in line with anticipated IME payment changes to manage this new system. CMS will require additional resources to assess institutions' performance and eligibility for incentive payments.

RECOMMENDATION 4-1

The Congress should authorize the secretary to change Medicare's funding of graduate medical education (gMe) to support the workforce skills needed in a delivery system that reduces cost growth while maintaining or improving quality.

- The secretary should establish the standards for distributing funds after consultation with representatives that include accrediting organizations, training programs, health care organizations, health care purchasers, patients, and consumers.

- The standards established by the secretary should, in particular, specify ambitious goals for practice- based learning and improvement, interpersonal and communication skills, professionalism, and systems- based practice, including integration of community- based care with hospital care.
- Performance-based GME funding under the new system should be allocated to an institution sponsoring gMe programs only if that institution met the new standards established by the secretary, and the level of funding would be tied to the institution's performance on the standards.

The indirect medical education (IME) payments above the empirically justified amount should be removed from the IMe adjustment and that sum would be used to fund the new performance-based gMe program. to allow time for the development of standards, the new performance-based gMe program should begin in three years (october 2013).

Rationale 4-1

Medicare's investment in GME should demand accountability for reaching specified standards and meeting the needs of high-value health systems. This new program would establish payment incentives that reward institutions—including teaching hospitals, medical schools, and other entities that may support residency programs—that meet specified educational goals and outcomes. Only those institutions meeting these specified criteria should be eligible for such incentive payments. Funding for this new program would come from a reduction in Medicare's IME payment—currently estimated to be twice the amount empirically attributable to higher patient care costs associated with a teaching environment.

Implications 4-1

Spending

- No Medicare program spending increase would occur; there would be some administrative costs.

Beneficiary and Provider

- There would be no direct impact on beneficiaries.
- Payments to individual teaching hospitals would increase or decrease, depending on their performance.

Improve collaboration between educators and teaching hospitals by increasing the transparency of medicare payments

During our examination of GME financing issues, some residency program directors voiced concerns that they have difficulty gaining information about their teaching hospitals' GME revenues because GME payments go directly to hospitals. Consequently, it can be challenging for them to judge whether Medicare's GME payments— as well as other revenues from other payers to support GME activities—are being distributed appropriately and equitably.

To improve information exchange between residency programs and provider institutions, Medicare could provide more transparent information on Medicare direct GME (DGME) and IME payments and hospital costs. This information, in the form of a short, public report, could prompt deliberations and collaborations among residency programs and hospitals about the distribution of these funds toward educational goals and community workforce needs. In addition, it would provide for greater public transparency in Medicare's role in supporting GME.

Specifically, the public report should include the following information, by institution:

- DGME revenues from Medicare
- IME revenues from Medicare
- number of residents counted by Medicare for direct GME payments
- number of residents counted by Medicare for IME payments
- Medicare's share of GME costs

Medicare could produce this information with little administrative burden, albeit with about a two-year lag. The payment information is already published by CMS on its website, but it is not necessarily in a user-friendly format or easy to find.[8] CMS could start producing these reports relatively quickly with the data it already has available. The institutions listed in these reports should include all those that received Medicare's DGME and IME funds in the reporting year.[9]

In response to a similar concern, New York State, in 2009, started requiring that residency training directors and teaching hospital administrators jointly submit an annual institutional budget for GME activities, reflecting both GME revenues and expenses, to the New York State Commissioner of Health.[10] This reporting is intended to foster greater dialogue between hospitals and their sponsoring institutions' designated academic affairs director to ensure that hospitals are aware of current and expected program needs and incorporate them into hospital budgets and that the academic affairs director is aware of how hospitals use these different sources of GME revenues.

Payment data

Payment data should include all DGME and IME payments that hospitals receive from Medicare, for both fee-for-service and Medicare Advantage. Also, for applicable institutions, this report should include relevant information on Medicare payments that support hospital- based nursing and other health professional training programs ($300 million in 2009).

Resident count data

The resident count data should be the count of residents used for Medicare DGME and IME payments. As the resident count used for DGME and IME payments can differ, separate DGME and IME resident counts need to be included in the report. Ideally, the report would also include data on the number of other types of health professionals that Medicare supports through its direct medical education payments for nursing and allied health professionals. The hospital cost reports, however, do not provide this level of detail; thus, a reporting mechanism would need to be developed to include such data.

Cost data

To make the cost data commensurate with the payment data, both DGME and IME costs reflecting Medicare's share of these expenses need to be reported. Although reporting Medicare payments and resident counts is relatively straightforward, some of the cost data are more complicated and would need to be computed. Medicare's report would need to cite issues concerning the accuracy and comparability of DGME cost data across providers (e.g., DGME cost data are not audited, hospitals may account for certain costs differently, and benefits hospitals receive from resident services are not reflected). Further work to refine, validate, and standardize the direct cost data may be necessary. Medicare could calculate and list IME costs as the institution's empirically justified share of Medicare IME revenues, but it would be important to also include caveats that these amounts are estimates that are based on national calculations and not reflective of a hospital's actual, specific indirect costs. Currently, hospitals do not compute hospital-specific IME costs. Although this approach would be an estimate, omitting any Medicare indirect costs from the report could leave the false impression that there are no indirect costs or that indirect costs equal the indirect payment.

Other issues

While this report would include both Medicare GME revenue and institutional cost information, it needs to make clear that these data cannot be used to perform a profit-and-loss analysis of GME activities. As noted above, there are a number of issues with the potential completeness and accuracy of the direct cost data and considerable uncertainty as to a hospital's actual indirect costs. Moreover, the financial benefits of residency training programs to the hospital and its physicians are not captured in these data; thus, any comparison of costs and revenues would provide an incomplete picture. We discuss these net financial impacts in a later section of this chapter related to Recommendation 4-4.

The proposed report would not divide payments and costs by specialty or list residents by specialty because these data are not readily available to Medicare. Nonetheless, residency program costs are likely to vary by specialty, as would their financial benefits to the hospital. Accordingly, some cross-subsidization is likely to occur across programs within an institution. Residency programs and hospitals would likely discuss this issue in their budgetary collaborations.

RECOMMENDATION 4-2

The secretary should annually publish a report that shows Medicare medical education payments received by each hospital and each hospital's associated costs. This report should be publicly accessible and clearly identify each hospital, the direct and indirect medical education payments received, the number of residents and other health professionals that Medicare supports, and Medicare's share of teaching costs incurred.

Rationale 4-2

Publication of this information is intended to prompt an informed dialogue between residency programs and hospitals on the resources that are required to support high-quality educational experiences for residents and fellows. It would also provide for greater public transparency on Medicare's role in supporting GME.

Implications 4-2

Spending

- No program spending increase would occur; there would be small administrative costs.

Beneficiary and Provider

- There would be no direct impact on beneficiaries.
- There would be no direct impact on providers.

Determine health workforce needs for a reformed delivery system

Medicare's payments for GME generally subsidize the specialty choices of both teaching hospitals (in their program offerings) and residents (in their career choices). As discussed earlier, these choices are strongly influenced by the payment rates of the services these specialties provide. The resulting physician mix of specialties is unlikely to ensure that the nation has an efficient supply of health professionals for well-functioning delivery systems.

For example, the share of third-year internal medicine residents choosing to practice primary care (rather than subspecialize or become hospitalists) has fallen from roughly 55 percent to 25 percent over the last decade (Figure 4-1).[11] Considering the significant financial investment that Medicare and other federal programs make in GME, a commitment to rigorous, independent workforce analysis is imperative to inform the most efficient use of these public funds. Such analysis should be conducted regularly to account for evolving clinical and health system factors.

Workforce studies are multifaceted, requiring not only creating projections of how many physicians, nurses, physician assistants, and others will be needed many years in the future but also what education and training the workforce will require. Some studies have projected there will be unmet demand unless the supply of physicians is greatly increased (Dill and Salsberg 2008); others have found current total numbers may be in the right range but specialty mix and geographic distribution issues may need adjustments (Mullan 2009); and still others find that efficient, high-quality systems can have lower physicianto-population ratios (Goodman 2004). The Bureau of Health Professions within HRSA periodically reports on health care workforce supply and demand issues, including physicians, nursing, and public health care workers, but these reports are not regularly updated.

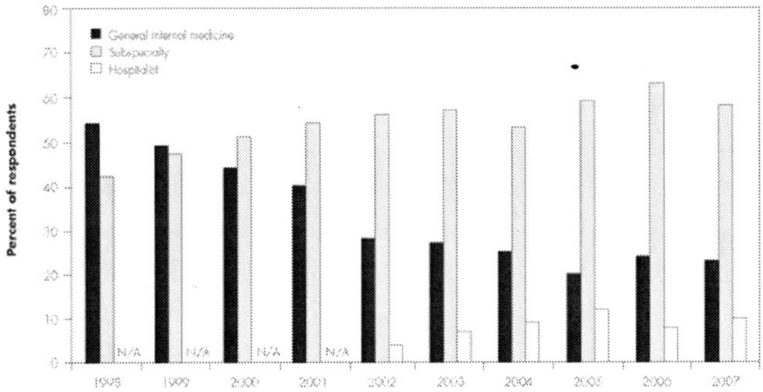

Note: N/A (not available).

Source: Bodenheimer, T. 2006. Primary care—Will it survive? The New England Journal of Medicine 355:861–864. Updated to include years 2006 and 2007, supplied by Thomas Bodenheimer, who obtained the relevant data from The American College of Physicians.

Figure 4-1. Proportions of third-year internal medical residents becoming specialists, subspecialists, and hospitalists are growing

The Commission strongly recommends that an analysis of our 21st century health care workforce needs be driven by the requirements of a high-value, affordable health care delivery system. In calculating benchmarks for physicians and specialty mix, this study should take into account successful examples of high-performing, integrated delivery systems (McCarthy and Mueller 2009).

Analyses that simply extrapolate demand projections based on current patterns of care could compromise the nation's chances of fostering a high-value health care system by producing increasing numbers of physicians who have a stake in the status quo. Alternatively, an improved delivery system will influence the total number of physicians needed in the workforce as well as the mix of professionals (e.g., the mix of primary care physicians, specialists, advanced practice nurses, and physician assistants).

Several existing workforce models assume the market is roughly in equilibrium in the base year. This assumption implies inefficiencies in current utilization and delivery patterns would transfer into the future (Bureau of Health Professions 2008). Even departures from the baseline in the models tend to assume only modest changes in the delivery system. A study is needed to assess how major improvements in the delivery system would affect the demand for physicians. If Medicare is unsustainable without delivery system reform, as the Commission maintains, a health care workforce that is consonant with a reformed delivery system is essential.

Recognizing the need for systematic health care workforce analysis, the Congress enacted several workforce and primary care provisions in the Patient Protection and Affordable Care Act of 2010 (PPACA) as described in a text box at the end of this chapter (p. 121). For example, the act establishes a National Health Workforce Commission tasked with examining workforce issues and charges HRSA's National Center for Health Care Workforce Analysis with data collection, analysis, and other reporting activities. The act also establishes state and regional centers for health workforce analysis to work in conjunction with this HRSA center. To carry out the workforce analyses that we recommend in this chapter, the Secretary could potentially collaborate with this new workforce commission and HRSA's workforce centers.

Recommendation 4-3

The secretary should conduct workforce analysis to determine the number of residency positions needed in the united states in total and by specialty. In addition, analysis should examine and consider the optimal level and mix of other health professionals. This work should be based on the workforce requirements of health care delivery systems that provide high-quality, high-value, and affordable care.

Rationale 4-3

Considering the investment that Medicare and other federal programs make in GME subsidies, a commitment to rigorous, independent workforce analysis is imperative to inform the most efficient use of these funds. Any change in the number of residents Medicare supports should be founded on an analysis of the health care workforce needs of a high-quality, high-value health care delivery system. Such an analysis should consider optimal care integration among physicians and other health professionals.

Implications 4-3

Spending

- No program spending increase would occur; there would be some administrative costs.

Beneficiary and Provider

- There would be no direct impact on beneficiaries.
- There would be no direct impact on providers.

Examine the net impact of residency program costs and benefits on hospitals' financial performance

Medicare's GME payment policies do not specifically consider the costs and benefits (together the net cost) of residency training programs or whether the net cost of training differs by specialty. IME payments, for instance, count all residents the same regardless of their experience. Although some broad-based payment differentials are built into the DGME payment rates—payments for primary care residents are slightly higher than for residents in other core specialties, and payments for subspecialty residents are set at half the rate for other residents—these payment differentials were the result of policy considerations and were not based on actual cost differences. The costs and benefits of sponsoring residency programs, however, are likely to vary significantly by specialty—potentially making certain specialty programs financially more attractive to an institution than others. Understanding how the net cost of training varies by specialty may help the Medicare program target its limited resources to support GME more effectively. Such an analysis would consider not only the net cost of training but also other factors, such as educational outcomes (see Recommendation 4-1) and the workforce needs of the health care system (see Recommendation 4-3). Determining the net costs of a given specialty residency training program will be challenging, as it is made up of a complex mix of educational expenses and potentially forgone revenues on the cost side and potentially increased patient care revenues and other effects on the benefit side. To date, there has been limited research on this issue.

Costs of supporting residency programs

Although residents' stipends are similar across specialties, the cost of supervising residents varies by specialty. For instance, not only do faculty salaries vary by specialty, but the opportunity cost of supervision (forgoing greater clinical productivity) also varies, depending on reimbursement levels for the hospitals' different service lines. Program administrative costs may also be higher for certain types of residencies in which training needs to be coordinated across multiple sites, supervision requirements are more intensive, or space needs are greater. Supervision costs are likely highest for first-year residents and fall as residents become more experienced. Indirect costs also may decline with increases in residents' experience, as more experienced residents likely have greater throughput (i.e., patient care productivity), order fewer unnecessary tests, and require less supervision.

Benefits of supporting residency programs

In addition to qualifying for higher payment rates, hospitals benefit from supporting residency programs in other ways—several of which vary by specialty. As part of their clinical education, residents provide services that otherwise would need to be provided by other health care professionals—often at higher wages (Rich et al. 2002). To the extent that certain types of services are more profitable for hospitals than others, residency programs in some specialties would offer more positive financial benefits than others. Additionally, in principle, more experienced residents should be able to perform services with greater independence and less supervision—resulting in a lower cost and greater benefit to the facility.

Another factor that may make some residency programs more attractive to teaching hospitals than others is their ability to draw in leaders in specialty fields that will enhance the prestige of the hospital and potentially lead to higher market share, patient volume, and revenues in select hospital departments. The value of resident services may also differ across settings, with hospital inpatient and outpatient departments potentially providing the highest return, as the services provided are generally reimbursed at higher rates. Given that a number of teaching hospitals train more residents than Medicare supports, some residency programs, particularly in subspecialties, may be financially self-sustaining. The Commission's analysis of Medicare data show, for instance, that hospitals that have exceeded the capped number of residents that Medicare subsidizes tend to have more subspecialty residents than those that are under the cap.[12] Also, the number and share of residents in subspecialties have grown (Salsberg et al. 2008).

In principle, Medicare's payments to institutions for resident education and training could reflect not only differences in performance but also differences in the net costs of supporting residency programs. While determining costs and benefits by specialty is complex, such research is needed to inform efficient distribution of Medicare GME funding.

RECOMMENDATION 4-4

The secretary should report to the Congress on how residency programs affect the financial performance of sponsoring institutions and whether residency programs in all specialties should be supported equally.

Rationale 4-4

The net impact that residency programs have on their hospitals' financial performance is likely to vary by specialty. Some residency programs may improve hospitals' financial performance (because of the ability to garner higher market share and be associated with higher revenue-producing services), while other residency programs may not. Although determining costs and benefits is a complex task, a better understanding of these financial impacts could inform a more efficient distribution of GME dollars among residency programs.

Implications 4-4

Spending

- No program spending increase would occur; there would be some administrative costs.

Beneficiary and Provider

- There would be no direct impact on beneficiaries.
- There would be no direct impact on providers.

Increase diversity among future physicians

Our June 2009 report discussed the underrepresentation of medical school students and residents from minority, lower income, and rural communities. Multiple research studies show that a diverse health care workforce is associated with better access to and quality of care for disadvantaged populations, greater patient choice and satisfaction, and better educational experience for students in health professions (Cooper et al. 2003, Health Resources and Services Administration 2006, Institute of Medicine 2004, Komaromy et al. 1996, Mertz and Grumbach 2001, Moy and Bartman 1995). Factors that increase the likelihood of students choosing careers in primary care and caring for underserved populations include being from a rural hometown and being an ethnic or racial minority (Brooks et al. 2002, Phillips et al. 2009).

Medicare's GME system is not able to address pipeline goals for increasing the economic, racial, or geographic diversity of the nation's physicians and other health professionals because Medicare's GME payments are focused on graduate-level physician training—much too late to influence individuals in their career choices. Interest in pursuing and preparing for careers in health professions (and specialty choices among those health professions) occurs along a continuum of stages in peoples' lives.

A number of HRSA programs are designed to recruit individuals—particularly from minority, rural, and low-income communities—into health careers. These programs (namely, those authorized by the Public Health Service Act, such as the National Health Service Corps (NHSC) and other programs under Title VII and Title VIII) include a variety of incentives, ranging from early education (grade school) programs to loan repayment programs. HRSA programs are also focused on promoting primary care access, particularly in underserved areas, and enhancing the cultural competence of this workforce by funding opportunities for medical students and residents to train in diverse settings and locations. These programs reach to a broader workforce than just physicians— including nurses, dentists, and other clinicians who focus on primary care. Recently, the PPACA reauthorized these HRSA programs and increased funding for several of them.

While the goals of these programs are on target with increasing the number and diversity of the nation's primary care workforce, and studies on selected HRSA programs find positive impacts, empirical research that comprehensively evaluates the longitudinal effectiveness of these programs is limited (Government Accountability Office 2006, Phillips et al. 2009, Rittenhouse et al. 2008). A more systematic approach for assessing impact across all programs is essential for determining the best way to invest resources to improve workforce diversity.

The Secretary should, therefore, complete a study that outlines a strategy for achieving specific goals related to workforce diversity in the nation's pipeline of health professionals. Potentially, this study could be conducted in collaboration with the new workforce Commission and HRSA workforce centers (mentioned earlier in this chapter) established by the PPACA. This study could also consider strategies that include partnerships with other federal departments, such as the Department of Education and the Department of Labor. Other important considerations in this study should be the need for both immediate and ongoing assessment of the effectiveness of HRSA's Title VII and Title VIII programs and to make available increased funding for the NHSC programs. Also, as recently recommended by the Advisory Committee on Training in Primary Care Medicine and Dentistry, HRSA should create a central data repository to collect and track information on HRSA program grantees (Advisory Committee on Training in Primary Care Medicine and Dentistry 2010).

Ultimately federal dollars that subsidize the nation's health care workforce should foster an optimal mix of clinicians—from different specialties, racial and ethnic backgrounds, rural and urban communities, and income levels—to achieve good access to a 21st century health care delivery system in all areas of the country. Determining the best strategy for reaching this objective should be a high priority to inform future spending decisions.

Summary of Health Workforce and Primary Care Provisions in the Patient Protection and Affordable Care Act of 2010

- Establishes a National Health Workforce Commission, which would report and make recommendations to the Congress and the Administration on the current state and projected needs of the U.S. health care workforce (Section 5101).
- Creates a competitive grant program for states to develop workforce planning strategies (Section 5102).
- Charges Health Resources and Services Administration's National Center for Health Care Workforce Analysis with data collection, analysis, and reporting on workforce programs and establishes state and regional centers for health workforce analysis (Section 5103).
- Reauthorizes and increases funding for several Public Health Service Act programs including Title VII and Title VIII, makes available increased funding for the National Health Service Corps, and establishes scholarship and loan repayment programs for a range of health care and public health professionals (Sections 5201 to 5207, and Sections 5308 to 5313).
- Establishes a primary care extension program through the Agency for Healthcare Research and Quality to educate primary care providers about preventive medicine, health promotion, chronic disease management, mental health service, and evidence-based therapies (Section 5405).
- Authorizes grants to geriatric education centers to support training for clinical faculty and family caregivers in geriatrics, chronic care management, and long-term care (Section 5305).
- Authorizes development grants and payments to support teaching health centers as community- based, ambulatory patient care centers

eligible for sponsoring physician residency programs in primary care (Section 5508).

- Directs the Secretary to redistribute 65 percent of currently unused residency slots and directs 75 percent of those slots for training primary care and general surgery and to states with the lowest resident physician-to-patient ratios, to states with the highest ratio of the population living in a health professional shortage area relative to the general population, and to states with rural hospitals (Section 5503).
- Modifies rules governing indirect medical education to promote resident training in ambulatory settings and in didactic and scholarly activities (Sections 5504 and 5505).
- Directs the Secretary to establish a demonstration program for hospitals to increase graduate nurse education training under Medicare (Section 5509).
- Provides a 10 percent payment bonus to primary care practitioners and general surgeons (pertains only to general surgeons in health professional shortage areas) for services provided under Medicare; makes Medicaid's payments for primary care services match Medicare's (Section 5501).
- Creates Center for Medicare and Medicaid Innovation to research, develop, test, and expand innovative payment and delivery service models, including the medical home (Section 3021).

RECOMMENDATION 4-5

The secretary should study strategies for increasing the diversity of our health professional workforce (e.g., increasing the shares from underrepresented rural, lower income, and minority communities) and report on what strategies are most effective to achieve this pipeline goal.

Rationale 4-5

Research has found that a diverse health care workforce is associated with better access to and quality of care for disadvantaged populations, greater patient choice and satisfaction, and better educational experience for students in health professions. Currently, Medicare's GME system is not designed to influence progress toward the goal of greater diversity among health professionals. A number of HRSA programs are designed to address relevant objectives under this goal, and research on specific programs shows some positive impacts, but comprehensive evaluation of these programs' longitudinal effectiveness is not well studied. An analysis that outlines a strategy for achieving specific health care workforce diversity goals and objectives is essential to optimize federal subsidies for this effort.

Implications 4-5

Spending

- No program spending increase would occur; there would be some administrative costs.

Beneficiary and Provider

- There would be no direct impact on beneficiaries.
- There would be no direct impact on providers.

References

[1] Advisory Committee on Training in Primary Care Medicine and Dentistry. (2010). Eighth annual report to the Secretary of the U.S. Department of Health and Human Services and to the U.S. Congress: *The redesign of primary care with implications for training*. Washington, DC: ACTPCMD.

[2] American College of Physicians. (2006). The impending collapse of primary care medicine and its implications for the state of the nation's health care. Washington, DC: ACP. January. http://www. acponline.o rg/advocacy. pdf.

[3] Association of American Medical Colleges. (2008). Diversity of U.S. medical students by parental income. *Analysis in brief, vol. 8*, no. 1. Washington, DC: AAMC.

[4] Blumenthal, D. (2002). Training tomorrow's doctors: *The medical education mission of academic health centers*. New York: Commonwealth Fund.

[5] Bodenheimer, T. (2006). Primary care—Will it survive? *New England Journal of Medicine*, *355*, no. 9 (August 31): 861-864.

[6] Boult, C., Counsell, S. R. & Leipzig, R. M., et al. (2010). Preparing primary care physicians to meet the geriatric imperative. *Health Affairs*. In press.

[7] Brooks, R. G., Walsh, M. & Mardon, R. E., et al. (2002). The roles of nature and nurture in the recruitment and retention of primary care physicians in rural areas: A review of the literature. *Academic Medicine*, *77*, no. 8 (August): 790-798.

[8] Bureau of Health Professions, Health Resources and Services Administration, Department of Health and Human Services. (2008). The physician workforce: *Projections and research into current issues affecting supply and demand. Rockville*, MD: Bureau of Health Professions.

[9] Byrne, C., Mercincavage, L. & Pan, E., et al. (2010). The value from investments in health information technology at the U.S. Department of Veterans Affairs. *Health Affairs*, 29, no. 4, 629-638.

[10]Chaudhry, S. I., Holmboe, E. & Beasley, B. W. (2008). The state of evaluation in internal medicine residency. *Journal of General Internal Medicine*, *23*, no. 7 (July): 1010-1015.

[11]Colwill, J. M., Cultice, J. M. & Kruse, R. L. (2008). Will generalist physician supply meet demands of an increasing and aging population? *Health Affairs*, *27*, no. 3 (May–June): w232-241.

[12]Congressional Budget Office. (2007). The health care system for veterans: *An interim report*. Washington, DC: CBO.

[13]Cooper, L. A., Roter, D. L. & Johnson, R. L., et al. (2003). Patient-centered communication, ratings of care, and concordance of patient and physician race. *Annals of Internal Medicine*, *139*, no. 11 (December 2): 907-915.

[14]Cordasco, K. M., Horta, M. & Lurie, N., et al. (2009). How are residency programs preparing our 21st century internists? A review of internal medicine residency programs' teaching on selected topics. *Contractor report prepared for MedPAC. Santa Monica*, CA: RAND Corporation.

[15]Council on Graduate Medical Education. (2007a). *COGME 18th report: New paradigms for physician training for improving access to health care*. Washington, DC: COGME. September.

[16]Council on Graduate Medical Education. (2007b). COGME 19th report: *Enhancing flexibility in graduate medical education*. Washington, DC: COGME.

[17]Dill, M. J. & Salsberg. E. S. (2008). *The complexities of physician supply and demand: Projections through 2025*. Washington, DC: Association of American Medical Colleges.

[18]Goodman, D. C. (2004). Do we need more physicians? *Health Affairs Web Exclusives* (January–June): W4-67-69.

[19]Government Accountability Office. (2006). Health professions education programs: *Action still needed to measure impact*. GAO–06–55. Washington, DC: GAO.

[20]Government Accountability Office. (2008). Primary care professionals: *Recent supply trends, projections, and valuation of services*. GAO–08–472T. Washington, DC: GAO.

[21]Health Resources and Services Administration, Department of Health and Human Services. (2006*). The rationale for diversity in the health professions: A review of the evidence*. Rockville, MD: HRSA. October. ftp://ftp.hrsa.gov/bhpr/workforce

[22]Holmboe, E. S., Bowen, J. L. & Green, M., et al. (2005). Reforming internal medicine residency training. A report from the Society of General Internal Medicine's task force for residency reform. *Journal of General Internal Medicine 20*, no. 12 (December): 1165-1172.

[23]Holmboe, E. S., Rodak, W. & Mills, G., et al. (2006). Outcomes-based evaluation in resident education: Creating systems and structured portfolios. *American Journal of Medicine*, *119*, no. 8 (August): 708-714.

[24]Institute of Medicine. (2008). Retooling for an aging America: *Building the health care workforce*. Washington, DC: National Academy Press.

[25]Komaromy, M., Grumbach, K. & Drake, M., et al. (1996). The role of black and Hispanic physicians in providing health care for underserved populations. *New England Journal of Medicine*, *334*, no. 20 (May 16), 1305-1310.

[26]Leipzig, R. M., Granville, L. & Simpson, D., et al. (2009). Keeping granny safe on July 1: A consensus on minimum geriatrics competencies for graduating medical students. *Academic Medicine*, *84*, no. 5 (May): 604-610.

[27]Lucien Leape Institute, National Patient Safety Foundation. (2010). Unmet needs: Teaching physicians to provide safe patient care. Boston, MA: *National Patient Safety Foundation*.

[28]Ludmerer, K. M. & Johns, M. M. (2005). Reforming graduate medical education. Journal *of the American Medical Association*, *294*, no. 9 (September 7), 1083-1087.

[29]McCarthy, D. & Mueller, K. (2009). Organizing for higher performance: Case studies of organized delivery systems. *Series overview, findings, and methods*. New York: Commonwealth Fund.

[30]Medicare Payment Advisory Commission. (2000). Report to the Congress: Medicare payment policy. Washington, DC: MedPAC.

[31]Medicare Payment Advisory Commission. (2009). Report to the Congress: *Improving incentives in the Medicare program*. Washington, DC: MedPAC.

[32]Medicare Payment Advisory Commission. (2010). Report to the Congress: *Medicare payment policy*. Washington, DC: MedPAC.

[33]Mullan, F. (2009). Workforce issues in health care reform: Assessing the present and preparing for the future. *Testimony before the Senate Finance Committee*. March 12.

[34]National Resident Matching Program. (2010). Advance data tables: 2010 *main residency match*.

[35]Papadakis, M. A., Arnold, G. K. & Blank, L. L., et al. 2008. Performance during internal medicine residency training and subsequent disciplinary action by state licensing boards. *Annals of Internal Medicine*, *148*, no. 11 (June 3), 869-876.

[36]Phillips, R. L., Dodoo, M. S. & Petterson, S., et al. (2009). Specialty and geographic distribution of the physician workforce: What influences medical student and resident choices? Prepared with support from the Josiah Macy, Jr., Foundation. Washington, DC: *The Robert Graham Center*.

[37]Rich, E. C., Liebow, M. & Srinivasan, M., et al. (2002). Medicare financing of graduate medical education. *Journal of General Internal Medicine*, 17, no. 4 (April), 283-292.

[38]Rittenhouse, D. R., Fryer, G. E. & Jr., Phillips, R. L., Jr., et al. (2008). Impact of Title VII training programs on community health center staffing and national health service corps participation. *Annals of Family Medicine*, *6*, no. 5 (September–October), 397-405.

[39]Salsberg, E., Rockey, P. H. & Rivers, K. L., et al. (2008). US residency training before and after the 1997 Balanced Budget Act. *Journal of the American Medical Association*, *300*, no. 10 (September 10), 1174-1180.

[40]Swensen, S. J., Meyer, G. S. & Nelson, E. C., et al. (2010). Cottage industry to postindustrial care—the revolution in health care delivery. *New England Journal of Medicine*, *362*, no. 5 (February 4), e12.

[41]Mertz, E. A. & Grumbach, K. (2001). Identifying communities with low dentist supply in California. *Journal of Public Health Dentistry*, *61*, no. 3 (Summer): 172-177.

[42]Meyers, F. J., Weinberger, S. E. & Fitzgibbons, J. P., et al. (2007). Redesigning residency training in internal medicine: The consensus report of the Alliance for Academic Internal Medicine Education Redesign Task Force. *Academic Medicine*, *82*, no. 12 (December), 1211-1219.

End Notes

[1] Although the Government Accountability Office found that the number of physician residents in primary care programs increased 6 percent over the last decade, research by Bodenheimer and colleagues suggests that an increasing share of these residents sought further subspecialty training or became hospitalists (Bodenheimer 2006, Government Accountability Office 2008). The number of family medicine residents increased by 3 percent for 2010 but decreased by the same percentage in 2009 (National Resident Matching Program 2010). This specialty has lower rates of subspecialization than internal medicine.

[2] Medicare also recognizes—for purposes of GME and IME funding—residency programs accredited by the American Dental Association and the Council on Podiatric Medical Education. ACGME also evaluates and accredits residency programs' institutional sponsors (mainly teaching hospitals) from an educational perspective.

[3] Specifically, ACGME reports that for the 2008–2009 academic year, 1 percent of residency programs had a "withdrawal of accreditation" status and fewer than 1 percent had a "probationary accreditation status." A more frequent action that ACGME takes when programs are not performing at high enough levels is to shorten the time between program evaluations.

[4] ACGME began to implement these outcome-based standards in 2001 and required full integration of them in residency programs beginning in 2006.

[5] ACGME-endorsed milestone projects are currently moving forward in internal medicine, pediatrics, general surgery, urology, ophthalmology, family medicine, and transitional year programs. Internal medicine, pediatrics, and general surgery have already defined milestones and are currently looking at ways to operationalize milestones in practice. Subspecialty societies like the American College of Cardiology and the American Gastroenterological Association are also developing milestones.

[6] With support from private foundations, the Association of American Medical Colleges, the American Medical Association, the Council of Medical Specialty Societies, and the American Geriatrics Society have launched a competency- based education and training initiative to ensure that all medical students and residents achieve basic competence in the care of older adults. The competencies, initially for graduating medical students, include measurable tasks associated with evidence-based geriatric care and patient safety. They fall into four main categories, those that: (1) are critical to patient safety and quality of care (medication management, self-care capacity, falls, balance and gait disorders, and hospital care for elders); (2) address the prevalence and underrecognition of cognitive impairment;

(3) address the complexity of diagnosis (atypical presentation of disease); and (4) address prioritizing care based on patient preference and function.

[7] Some have raised concerns, however, that promoting more nonhospital residency experience is less relevant for Medicare GME policies because the share of Medicare patients in many of these settings is smaller.

[8] See http://www.cms.hhs.gov/CostReports/02_ HospitalCostReport.asp#TopOfPage.

[9] In the future, the report could also include federally qualified health centers, rural health clinics, teaching health centers (established in the Patient Protection and Affordable Care Act of 2010), and other places that receive Medicare or other federal support to cover direct and indirect costs of residency training programs. Data for such training sites, however, would need to come from sources other than the Medicare cost reports.

[10] The initial idea for a joint budget came from the New York Council on Graduate Medical Education, which recommended that these budgets should be generated by individual residency program directors for the hospital leadership team. With one year of reporting completed, the comparability of expense data across providers has proven somewhat problematic as not all GME expenses, such as those made for malpractice and simulation laboratories, are accounted for in the same way across institutions.

[11] Although the Government Accountability Office found that the number of physician residents in primary care programs increased 6 percent over the last decade, Figure 4-1 suggests that many of these residents sought further subspecialty training or became hospitalists (Government Accountability Office 2008). The number of family medicine residents increased by 3 percent for 2010 but decreased by the same percentage in 2009 (National Resident Matching Program 2010). This specialty has lower rates of subspecialization than internal medicine.

[12] Medicare caps the number of residents a hospital can count for direct and indirect GME payments at 1996 levels. There are also certain subspecialties that do not have ACGME accreditation that train fellows, but hospitals receive no direct GME or IME payments for these residents (e.g., gynecologic oncology, reproductive endocrinology and infertility), providing further evidence that some residency programs may be self-sustaining.

CHAPTER SOURCES

The following chapters have been previously published:

Chapter 1 – This is an edited, excerpted and augmented edition of a Rand Health publication, Number 09-5, dated July 2009.

Chapter 2 – This is an edited, excerpted and augmented edition of a Medpac Report to the Congress, dated June 2009.

Chapter 3 – This is an edited, excerpted and augmented edition of a Medpac Report to the Congress, dated June 2010.

INDEX

C

D

E

F

L

M

N

O

P

Q

R